1001 MCQs to Master
Addiction Medicine

1001 MCQs to Master
Addiction Medicine

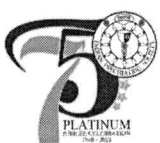

Indian Psychiatric Society Publication

Editors
Shahul Ameen MD
Consultant Psychiatrist
St Thomas Hospital
Changanacherry, Kerala, India

Anil Kakunje DPM MD
Professor and Head
Department of Psychiatry
Yenepoya Medical College, Deralakatte
Mangaluru, Karnataka, India

Sai Krishna Tikka DPM MD
Associate Professor
Department of Psychiatry
All India Institute of Medical Sciences
Bibinagar, Hyderabad, Telangana, India

Snehil Gupta MD DNB
Associate Professor
Department of Psychiatry
All India Institute of Medical Sciences
Bhopal, Madhya Pradesh, India

Mrugesh Vaishnav MD
Director
Samvedana Happiness Hospital
Ahmedabad, Gujarat, India

Foreword
Pratima Murthy

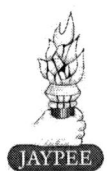

JAYPEE BROTHERS MEDICAL PUBLISHERS
The Health Sciences Publisher
New Delhi | London

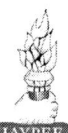 **Jaypee Brothers Medical Publishers (P) Ltd**

Headquarters
Jaypee Brothers Medical Publishers (P) Ltd
EMCA House, 23/23-B
Ansari Road, Daryaganj
New Delhi 110 002, India
Landline: +91-11-23272143, +91-11-23272703
+91-11-23282021, +91-11-23245672
Email: jaypee@jaypeebrothers.com

Corporate Office
Jaypee Brothers Medical Publishers (P) Ltd
4838/24, Ansari Road, Daryaganj
New Delhi 110 002, India
Phone: +91-11-43574357
Fax: +91-11-43574314
Email: jaypee@jaypeebrothers.com

Overseas Office
JP Medical Ltd
83 Victoria Street, London
SW1H 0HW (UK)
Phone: +44 20 3170 8910
Fax: +44 (0)20 3008 6180
Email: info@jpmedpub.com

Website: www.jaypeebrothers.com
Website: www.jaypeedigital.com

© 2024, Jaypee Brothers Medical Publishers and Indian Psychiatric Society

The views and opinions expressed in this book are solely those of the original contributor(s)/author(s) and do not necessarily represent those of editor(s) or publisher of the book.

All rights reserved. No part of this publication may be reproduced, stored or transmitted in any form or by any means, electronic, mechanical, photocopying, recording or otherwise, without the prior permission in writing of the publishers.

All brand names and product names used in this book are trade names, service marks, trademarks or registered trademarks of their respective owners. The publisher is not associated with any product or vendor mentioned in this book.

Medical knowledge and practice change constantly. This book is designed to provide accurate, authoritative information about the subject matter in question. However, readers are advised to check the most current information available on procedures included and check information from the manufacturer of each product to be administered, to verify the recommended dose, formula, method and duration of administration, adverse effects and contraindications. It is the responsibility of the practitioner to take all appropriate safety precautions. Neither the publisher nor the author(s)/editor(s) assume any liability for any injury and/or damage to persons or property arising from or related to use of material in this book.

This book is sold on the understanding that the publisher is not engaged in providing professional medical services. If such advice or services are required, the services of a competent medical professional should be sought.

Every effort has been made where necessary to contact holders of copyright to obtain permission to reproduce copyright material. If any have been inadvertently overlooked, the publisher will be pleased to make the necessary arrangements at the first opportunity.

Inquiries for bulk sales may be solicited at: jaypee@jaypeebrothers.com

1001 MCQs to Master Addiction Medicine

First Edition: **2024**, Reprint 2025

ISBN: 978-93-5696-573-7

Printed in India

Contributors

Amit Singh DM (Addiction Psychiatry)
Assistant Professor
Department of Psychiatry
King George Medical University
Lucknow, Uttar Pradesh, India
Email: amitsingh0612@gmail.com

Aniruddha Basu
MBBS MD PDF (Addiction Medicine) DM (Addiction Psychiatry)
Associate Professor
Department of Psychiatry
All India Institute of Medical Sciences
Kalyani, West Bengal, India
Email: aniruddha.psy@aiimskalyani.edu.in

Aniruddha Mukherjee MD (Psychiatry)
Professor
Department of Psychiatry
Center for Addiction Psychiatry
Central Institute of Psychiatry
Ranchi, Jharkhand, India
Email: dr_aniruddha@hotmail.com

Ankita Chattopadhyay
MBBS MD (Psychiatry) DNB (Psychiatry) DM (Addiction Psychiatry)
Assistant Professor
Department of Psychiatry
JIPMER
Puducherry, India
Email: chattopadhyayankita@gmail.com

Anuradha Moirangthem
MD (Psychiatry)
Senior Resident
Department of Psychiatry
Regional Institute of Medical Sciences
Imphal, Manipur, India
Email: dr.anuradha.moirangthem@gmail.com

Arghya Pal MD DNB
Assistant Professor
Department of Psychiatry
All India Institute of Medical Sciences
Raebareli, Uttar Pradesh, India
Email: drarghyamb@gmail.com

Arpit Parmar
MD (Psychiatry) DM (Addiction Psychiatry)
Associate Professor
Department of Psychiatry
All India Institute of Medical Sciences
Bhubaneswar, Odisha, India
Email: dr.arpitparmar@gmail.com

Aworshim Muivah
MD (Psychiatry)
Senior Resident
Department of Psychiatry
Regional Institute of Medical Sciences
Imphal, Manipur, India
Email: shimmuivah913@gmail.com

Dhrubajyoti Bhuyan
MD (Psychiatry)
Associate Professor
Department of Psychiatry
Assam Medical College
Dibrugarh, Assam, India
Email: dr.dhrubajyoti@gmail.com

Gayatri Bhatia
MD DM (Addiction Psychiatry)
Assistant Professor
Department of Psychiatry
All India Institute of Medical Sciences
Rajkot, Gujarat, India
Email: gayatribhatia90@gmail.com

Contributors

Jayant Mahadevan
MD (Psychiatry) DM (Addiction Psychiatry)
Assistant Professor
Department of Psychiatry
Center for Addiction Medicine
National Institute of Mental Health and Neurosciences
Bengaluru, Karnataka, India
Email: jayantmahadevan@gmail.com

Manmeet Kaur Brar
MBBS MD (Psychiatry) DM (Addiction Psychiatry)
Senior Resident
Department of Psychiatry
National Drug Dependence Treatment Center
All India Institute of Medical Sciences
New Delhi, India
Email: mksidhu27@gmail.com

Mohita Joshi
MD (Psychiatry) PDF in Addiction Medicine
Senior Resident
Department of Psychiatry
King George Medical University
Lucknow, Uttar Pradesh, India
Email: mohitajoshi123@gmail.com

Mona Nongmeikapam MD (Psychiatry)
Assistant Professor
Department of Psychiatry
Regional Institute of Medical Sciences
Imphal, Manipur, India
Email: mona_nk1@yahoo.co.in

Nandhini Bojappen
MD (Psychiatry) PDF in Addiction Medicine
Senior Resident
Department of Psychiatry
Center for Addiction Medicine
National Institute of Mental Health and Neurosciences
Bengaluru, Karnataka, India
Email: drnandhinibojappen@gmail.com

Preethy Kathiresan
MBBS MD (Psychiatry) DNB (Psychiatry)
DM (Addiction Psychiatry)
Assistant Professor
Department of Psychiatry
All India Institute of Medical Sciences
New Delhi, India
Email: princyaiims@gmail.com

Rahul Mathur
MD DNB (Psychiatry)
Senior Resident
Department of Psychiatry
All India Institute of Medical Sciences
New Delhi, India
Email: rahul17.aiims@gmail.com

Rashmi Chakraborty
MBBS MD
Senior Resident
Department of Psychiatry
All India Institute of Medical Sciences
Kalyani, West Bengal, India
Email: drparamitachak@gmail.com

Senjam Gojendra Singh
MD (Psychiatry)
Associate Professor and Head
Department of Psychiatry
Regional Institute of Medical Sciences
Imphal, Manipur, India
Email: drgojendra@gmail.com

Siddharth Sarkar
MD (Addiction Psychiatry)
Additional Professor
Department of Psychiatry
National Drug Dependence Treatment Center
All India Institute of Medical Sciences
New Delhi, India
Email: sidsarkar22@gmail.com

Sourav Khanra
MD (Psychiatry) DNB (Psychiatry)
Associate Professor
Department of Psychiatry
Center for Addiction Psychiatry
Central Institute of Psychiatry
Ranchi, Jharkhand, India
Email: souravpsy@gmail.com

Sukriti Mukherjee MBBS MD
Senior Resident
Department of Psychiatry
All India Institute of Medical Sciences
Kalyani, West Bengal, India
Email: mukherjeesukriti@gmail.com

Tanmay Joshi
MD (Psychiatry) DM (Addiction Psychiatry)
Assistant Professor
Department of Psychiatry
All India Institute of Medical Sciences
Bhopal, Madhya Pradesh, India
Email: tanmayjoshi89@gmail.com

Tathagata Mahintamani
DPM DNB (Psychiatry) DM (Addiction Psychiatry)
Assistant Professor
Department of Psychiatry
LGBRIMH
Tezpur, Assam, India
Email: mahintamani@gmail.com

Foreword

The field of addiction is growing rapidly. There has been an explosive surge in understanding of the biological mechanisms of addiction and its effects on the brain and other bodily systems. Epidemiological transitions in the patterns of substance use have occurred much more rapidly in the increasingly 'flat' new world. Just as you think you have grasped the basic understanding of existing drugs of abuse and addictions, newer and 'designer' drugs emerge; or older drugs rediscovered for their addictive potential come to light. Newer technologies to detect drugs of abuse and contemporary investigations to assess their impact on the human body, through imaging, ultrasound, epigenetics and several other investigative modalities demands that the clinician constantly learns, unlearns and relearns facts about addiction. Appropriate pharmacological treatment of acute conditions, as well as relapse prevention, requires a good knowledge of both pharmacotherapy of individual drugs as well as their interactions, particularly in conditions with co-morbidity and multi-morbidity. The medico-legal dimension adds further complexity, as do different policy approaches across the globe. Many psychosocial approaches to substance use have now been empirically validated. A host of brief and intensive psychotherapeutic approaches have been evaluated for addictive disorders and more recently, the interest and testing of evidence for digital interventions in the field is growing. The universe of addiction has also expanded to include a wide range of behavioral addictions. Further, there has been expanding knowledge on proximal and distal risk factors for addiction, ranging from genetic and familial risks to environmental risks. Thus, trainees need to keep abreast of both stable facts as well as changes in the substance use and addiction scenario in our context.

Solving multiple choice questions (MCQs) is one way to update oneself regarding the current science and art of managing addictive disorders. Well-constructed MCQs are a quick and efficient way to update information across a wide area, and enable easy recall. MCQs incorporating clinical vignettes can also provide important management tips in clinical situations. The wide range of topics covered in MCQs can also spur the reader to read more about the topic that is being addressed. It is important of course to underscore that MCQs need to be complimented with a deeper understanding of the topic and cannot be a substitute for higher order learning and gaining of clinical skills.

Foreword

I congratulate the Indian Psychiatric Society (IPS) publication committee, the contributors and editors of the 1001 MCQs to Master Addiction Medicine for so thoughtfully compiling these MCQs comprehensively covering diverse areas of addictions and hope this will be a valuable guide to trainees in both psychiatry, related postgraduate disciplines as well as undergraduate medical students.

Pratima Murthy
Director and Senior Professor of Psychiatry
National Institute of Mental Health and Neurosciences
Bengaluru, Karnataka, India

Message

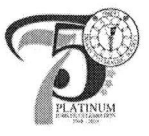 **Indian Psychiatric Society**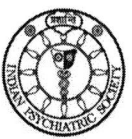

All professional organizations have a pleasant duty to address the needs of the younger generation, especially students. The Indian Psychiatric Society has always tried to contribute in this area. Establishing a publication subcommittee is a comparatively new initiative. Though we commenced commercial publication just 6 years ago, by now we have a catalogue of about two dozen books. In this catalogue, there are many handy, readable, and affordable publications that were badly needed.

1001 MCQs to Master Addiction Medicine is also one of them. All sub-disciplines of psychiatry are important. However, to date, only three are super-specialties and addiction psychiatry is one of them. This highlights the importance of in-depth knowledge in this area. I am sure the MCQ book will not only help the readers pass entrance tests but also inspire them.

We are proud of our publication committee led by Dr Anil Kakunje for the highly productive year and congratulate the editors and authors for this very useful book.

We express sincere thanks to Jaypee Brothers Medical Publishers, especially, Ms Chetna Malhotra (Senior Director—Professional Publishing, Marketing and Business Development) and Pragati Singh (Development Editor) for producing the book in an exceptional manner.

Vinay Kumar	**Laxmikant Rathi**	**Arabinda Brahma**
President	Vice President	Hon. General Secretary

Preface

Since its inception, the Publication Committee of the Indian Psychiatric Society has been creative and innovative in finding topics to prepare books. Early last year, when the current Committee had its first online meeting, one of the suggestions was for MCQ books on superspecialty topics. The major intention was to fill the void that those preparing for DM entrance do not have any MCQ books to check their knowledge or get the latest information in an MCQ format. That is how the idea for this book was born. We also felt that, besides DM aspirants, books like this would benefit those preparing for the NEET PG exam and practicing psychiatrists who want to brush up their knowledge and update themselves about the recent developments in the field.

We thank the Indian Psychiatric Society (IPS) office Bearers, Drs Vinay Kumar (President), Arabinda Brahma (Hon. General Secretary), OP Singh (Hon. Editor), M Aleem Siddiqui (Hon. Treasurer), and Laxmikant Rathi (Vice President) for their support to the Publication Committee in general and this book in particular.

All the authors we chose promptly agreed to build a team and prepare the chapters at short notice, though writing in this format is not something we commonly do. They all submitted the chapters within the deadline, making it possible to release the book at ANCIPS 2024. They were inventive and meticulous in preparing diverse questions, incorporating clinical vignettes, including the most recent information about topics ranging from neurobiology to Indian laws, etc. They were very cooperative about the revision process, too. They deserve a standing ovation from all of us.

As usual, the dynamic team at Jaypee Brothers Medical Publishers was quick and efficient in converting the accepted chapters to the book format. Our appreciation goes to Ms Chetana Malhotra (Senior Director—Professional Publishing, Marketing and Business Development), and Ms Pragati Singh (Development Editor) for their efforts in creating this book in a timely and professional manner.

Also, we would like to thank Sreya Mariyam Salim for the cover image.

Shahul Ameen
Anil Kakunje
Sai Krishna Tikka
Snehil Gupta
Mrugesh Vaishnav

Contents

1. **Alcohol** 1
   Nandhini Bojappen, Mohita Joshi, Jayant Mahadevan

2. **Nicotine** 35
   Preethy Kathiresan, Ankita Chattopadhyay, Tanmay Joshi

3. **Cannabis** 50
   Rashmi Chakraborty, Sukriti Mukherjee, Aniruddha Basu

4. **Opioids** 77
   Amit Singh, Arpit Parmar, Rahul Mathur

5. **Stimulants, Caffeine, and Inhalants** 91
   Siddharth Sarkar, Dhrubajyoti Bhuyan, Manmeet Kaur Brar

6. **Hallucinogens, Phencyclidine, and Methylenedioxymethamphetamine** 107
   Arpit Parmar, Amit Singh, Arghya Pal

7. **Hypnotics and Prescription Drug Abuse** 121
   Sourav Khanra, Aniruddha Mukherjee, Tathagata Mahintamani

8. **Gambling, Gaming, and Other Behavioral Addictions** 137
   *Senjam Gojendra Singh, Mona Nongmeikapam,
   Anuradha Moirangthem, Aworshim Muivah*

9. **Miscellaneous** 158
   Gayatri Bhatia, Ankita Chattopadhyay, Rahul Mathur

CHAPTER 1

Alcohol

Nandhini Bojappen, Mohita Joshi, Jayant Mahadevan

1. According to the National Survey on Extent and Patterns of Drug Use (2019), the prevalence of the problem of alcohol use in the general population between the ages of 10 and 75 years was:
   a. 15.2%
   b. 10.8%
   c. 5.2%
   d. 1.5%

2. According to the National Survey on Extent and Patterns of Drug Use (2019), the prevalence of current alcohol use at 35.6% was the highest in:
   a. Kerala
   b. Punjab
   c. Goa
   d. Chhattisgarh

3. According to the National Survey on Extent and Patterns of Drug Use (2019), the most commonly used beverages by current alcohol users are:
   a. Spirits > Wine > Light beer > Strong beer
   b. Strong beer > Spirits > Light beer > Wine
   c. Spirits > Strong beer > Light beer > Wine
   d. Spirits > Light beer > Strong Beer > Wine

4. GENACIS (Gender, alcohol, and culture: An International Study) was a multidisciplinary, international project which included India as one of the sites. It aimed to study:
   a. Gender, age, and cannabis
   b. Genetics, alcohol, and cannabis
   c. Gender, alcohol, and culture
   d. Genetics, alcohol, and culture

5. The partition coefficient for ethanol between blood and alveolar air is about:
   a. 500:1
   b. 1,150:1
   c. 2,100:1
   d. 3,500:1

6. Peak blood levels of ethanol usually occur:
   a. 30–60 minutes after ingestion on an empty stomach
   b. 10–15 minutes after ingestion on an empty stomach
   c. 30–60 minutes after ingestion on a full stomach
   d. 10–15 minutes after ingestion on a full stomach

Alcohol

7. Ethanol metabolism in the liver is associated with all of the following, *except*:
   a. Accumulation of lactate
   b. Reduced activity of the tricarboxylic acid cycle
   c. Accumulation of acetyl-CoA (coenzyme A)
   d. Reduction in fatty acid synthesis and depletion of triacylglycerides

8. The hepatic enzyme that accounts for about 10% of the metabolism of alcohol is:
   a. Aldehyde dehydrogenase (ALDH)
   b. Alcohol dehydrogenase (ADH)
   c. CYP2E1
   d. Catalase

9. Which of the following statements is TRUE about the enzyme ADH?
   a. It typically exhibits zero-order kinetics
   b. It converts acetaldehyde to acetate
   c. Women have higher levels of ADH compared to men
   d. It is inhibited by disulfiram

10. Heritability of alcohol use disorder (AUD) based on twin studies is:
    a. 70–80
    b. 10–20
    c. 40–60
    d. 100

11. With regards to the genetics of AUD, all of the following are true, *except*:
    a. ALDH2*2 allele is associated with flushing, tachycardia, and nausea upon consumption of small amounts of alcohol as it reduces acetaldehyde dehydrogenase activity
    b. Asn40Asp variation of the *OPRM1* gene is associated with therapeutic response to acamprosate in patients with AUD
    c. DRD2-Taq1A polymorphism has been noted to have a small but significant association with AUD
    d. Polymorphisms in the ADH gene and its subtypes have been most consistently reported in genome-wide association studies of AUD

12. The genetic polymorphisms found to be protective from AUD among East Asians are:
    a. ADH1B*2 and ALDH2*2
    b. ADH1B*3 and ALDH1*1
    c. GABRA2
    d. ADH2 and ALDH1*1

13. The genetic polymorphism associated with increased risk of esophageal cancer among individuals who consume alcohol is:
    a. ALDH2*2
    b. ALDH1*1
    c. ADH1B*2
    d. ADH1B*3

14. Acute ethanol ingestion is associated with an enhancement in the activity of all of the following ligand- and voltage-gated ion channels, *except*:
    a. Gamma-aminobutyric acid subtype A (GABA$_A$) receptor-operated channels
    b. Glycine receptor-operated channels
    c. N-methyl-D-aspartate (NMDA) receptor-operated channels
    d. Nicotinic acetylcholine (ACh) receptor-operated channels

15. All of the following statements are TRUE about alcohol and GABA, *except*:
    a. GABA$_A$ receptors that contain ρ subunit are inhibited by alcohol
    b. GABA$_A$ receptors that contain the δ subunit possess high sensitivity to relatively low levels of alcohol
    c. GABA$_A$ receptors that contain γ2L subunit are important for alcohol potentiation of channel function in some studies
    d. GABA$_A$ knock-out and knock-in mice show significant changes in alcohol-induced behaviors, emphasizing the central role of GABA$_A$ receptors

16. The following is TRUE about alcohol and glutamate:
    a. NMDA receptors expressed in most neurons are readily potentiated by alcohol at concentrations (10–100 mM)
    b. Activation of NMDA receptors in the prefrontal cortex may underlie some of the cognitive deficits and errors in judgment observed during alcohol intoxication
    c. Chronic exposure to alcohol increases the density and clustering of NMDA but not non-NMDA glutamate receptors
    d. Antagonism of NMDA receptors may lead to negative reinforcement of alcohol use behaviors

17. All of the following statements are TRUE about preclinical findings related to treatments for AUD, *except*:
    a. Long-acting dopamine agonist, bromocriptine administered systemically, shifts a rat's preference from alcohol to water, especially in those strains of rats that show alcohol preference
    b. In mice, ivermectin, a positive allosteric modulator of P2X4 channel function, reduces ethanol consumption in various drinking models
    c. Enhancing SK channel activity in the nucleus accumbens with an allosteric modulator (chlorzoxazone) increased alcohol consumption in rats
    d. 5HT3 receptor antagonists such as ondansetron block the rat's ability to discriminate ethanol from saline, decreasing alcohol consumption

18. Behavioral tolerance of alcohol is described as follows:
    a. A person learns through practice how to perform tasks effectively while experiencing the effects of alcohol
    b. Adaptations of alcohol metabolizing systems to rid the body of alcohol more rapidly
    c. An adaptation of the nervous system so that it can function despite high blood alcohol concentrations (BACs) by resisting the actions of alcohol on the cell
    d. Experiencing the same effect with a lower concentration of substance

19. Which of the following statements about the definition of hazardous alcohol use is FALSE?
    a. In the US, consumption of >14 units of alcohol by men in a week is considered hazardous
    b. In the UK, consuming >7 units of alcohol by women in a week is considered hazardous
    c. In the US, consumption of >7 units of alcohol by women in a week is considered hazardous
    d. In pregnancy and children below the age of 16, any alcohol use is hazardous

20. As per the National Institute of Alcohol and Alcoholism (NIAAA), binge drinking is defined as:
    a. A pattern of drinking alcohol that brings BAC to 0.08% or 0.08 g of alcohol per deciliter or higher
    b. Consumption of two or more drinks for women or three or more drinks for men within about 2 hours
    c. Consumption of four or more drinks for women or five or more drinks for men within 24 hours
    d. Pattern of drinking alcohol that brings BAC to 0.04% or 0.04 g of alcohol per deciliter or higher

21. All of the following are screening tools used for AUDs, *except*:
    a. AUDIT (Alcohol Use Disorders Identification Test)
    b. CAGE (Cut down, Annoyed, Guilty, and Eye-opener)
    c. MAST (Michigan Alcoholism Screening Test)
    d. SADQ (Severity of Alcohol Dependence Questionnaire)

22. Expand CAGE, which is a common screening tool used for alcohol use in general medical settings:
    a. Cut down, Annoyance, Guilt, Eye-opener
    b. Craving, Annoyance, Guilt, Eye-opener
    c. Cut down, Annoyance, Grandiosity, Eye-opener
    d. Cut down, Anxiety, Guilt, Eye-opener

23. AUDIT-C (consumption) consists of all of the following items, *except*:
    a. Quantity of alcohol use
    b. Frequency of alcohol use
    c. Frequency of heavy alcohol use
    d. Consequences of alcohol use

24. With regards to the AUDIT, the correct statement is:
    a. The AUDIT consists of a total of 15 items
    b. The AUDIT assesses alcohol intake, alcohol dependence, and alcohol-related harm
    c. A score of >20 on the AUDIT is the cutoff for hazardous or harmful use
    d. The AUDIT is a commonly used diagnostic tool for identifying AUDs

25. The Clinical Institute Withdrawal Assessment of Alcohol Scale, Revised (CIWA-Ar) is commonly used to assess the severity of alcohol withdrawal. All of the following are TRUE about it, *except*:
    a. A score of 11–15 for moderate withdrawal
    b. Scores >15 may need an intensive care setting
    c. Consists of 10 questions
    d. All questions can be applied to patients with delirium tremens (DT)

26. All of the following tools assess the patient's level of motivation related to alcohol use, *except*:
    a. Readiness to change questionnaire
    b. Stages of change readiness and treatment eagerness scale
    c. University of Rhode Island Change Assessment
    d. Alcohol abstinence self-efficacy scale

27. All of the following are TRUE about blood alcohol testing, *except*:
    a. Testing for alcohol levels in the blood can be done using enzymatic analysis or gas chromatography of the headspace
    b. Specimens for venipuncture should be drawn using an alcohol-free antiseptic
    c. High acetone levels, such as those in diabetic ketoacidosis or starvation, can be metabolized to isopropanol and mask ethanol levels measured by enzymatic analysis
    d. Gas chromatography is the gold standard for measuring ethanol in forensic laboratories

28. All of the following are direct metabolites of ethanol which may be detected in the laboratory, *except*:
    a. Ethyl glucuronide
    b. Carbohydrate deficient transferrin

6 Alcohol

c. Ethyl sulfate
d. Fatty acid ethyl ester

29. The following statements are TRUE about ethyl glucuronide:
    a. It is a phase I metabolite of ethanol
    b. It is a major metabolite of ethanol and comprises 10% of its total elimination
    c. It can be detected in postmortem body fluids and tissues
    d. Mouthwashes or alcohol-containing hand sanitizing gels do not elevate their levels

30. All of the following are TRUE regarding the effects of alcohol intoxication, *except*:
    a. At a blood ethanol concentration (BEC) in the range of 20–99 mg%, loss of muscular coordination begins, and changes in mood, personality, and behavior occur
    b. Neurological impairment occurs at a BEC range of 100–199 mg%, accompanied by prolonged reaction time, ataxia, incoordination, and mental impairment
    c. Hypothermia may occur at a BEC range of 200–299 mg%, along with severe dysarthria and amnesia, with stage I anesthesia
    d. In very young and naïve drinkers, BECs of 300 mg% may be associated with coma and death, especially when levels are reached quickly

31. The most common reason for respiratory depression in a patient with alcohol intoxication is:
    a. Coingestion of other central nervous system (CNS) depressants such as opioids and benzodiazepines (BDZs)
    b. BEC of 200 mg/dL
    c. Diagnosis of acute alcoholic hepatitis
    d. Presence of thiamine deficiency

32. Which of the following is an agent which is seen to enhance the metabolic clearance of alcohol and speed recovery of intoxicated individuals?
    a. Naltrexone
    b. Fomepizole
    c. Metadoxine
    d. Acamprosate

33. About blackouts related to alcohol use, the following statement is TRUE:
    a. It is an anterograde amnesia for the period when a person was drinking heavily but remained awake
    b. It is identical in presentation to a similar state occurring with all drugs of abuse

c. It is a very rare phenomenon seen in <1% of drinkers in their lifetime
d. It is a loss of consciousness while drinking alcohol

34. A 28-year-old man developed a hangover after a night of heavy drinking. All of the following are TRUE about this condition, *except*:
    a. The effect of intermediate products of ethanol metabolism, congeners and by-products of individual alcohol preparations contribute to the occurrence of a hangover
    b. Dehydration, electrolyte imbalance, disruption of sleep and other biological rhythms, and increased physical activity while intoxicated contribute to a hangover
    c. Patients with hangover have a diffuse slowing on electroencephalography (EEG) persisting up to 16 hours after blood alcohol levels become undetectable
    d. Dark liquors, such as brandy and whiskey, appear to be associated with a reduced hangover frequency and severity

35. As per DSM-5 (Diagnostic and Statistical Manual of Mental Disorders, Fifth Edition), the number of criteria that need to be met to fulfil a diagnosis of moderate AUD are:
    a. 2–3
    b. 4–5
    c. 6–7
    d. >8

36. As per DSM-5, early remission in AUD is defined as:
    a. None of the criteria for AUD (except craving) has been met for at least 3 months but <12 months
    b. None of the criteria for AUD (except craving) has been met for at least 6 months but <12 months
    c. None of the criteria for AUD (except craving) has been met for at least 1 month but <12 months
    d. None of the criteria for AUD (except craving) has been met for at least 12 months

37. The ICD-11 (International Classification of Diseases 11th Revision) criteria for early full remission and sustained full remission in describing the course of alcohol dependence are:
    a. Early full remission is 1–12 months; sustained full remission is >12 months
    b. Early full remission is 3–12 months; sustained full remission is >12 months
    c. Early full remission is 1–12 months; sustained full remission is >24 months
    d. Early full remission is 3–12 months; sustained full remission is >24 months

38. All of the following alcohol-induced psychiatric conditions are described in ICD-11, *except*:
    a. Alcohol-induced psychotic disorder
    b. Alcohol-induced mood disorder
    c. Alcohol-induced anxiety disorder
    d. Alcohol-induced impulse control disorder

39. All of the following are TRUE about alcohol-induced psychotic disorder, *except*:
    a. It should not be exclusively part of the course of delirium
    b. Symptoms must persist for a substantial period (>6 months) after cessation of withdrawal/intoxication
    c. Associated with delusions, hallucinations, or both
    d. Symptoms typically begin during or soon after alcohol intoxication or withdrawal

40. The TRUE statement about alcohol-induced depressive disorder is:
    a. It is less prevalent than major depressive disorder (MDD) in patients with alcohol dependence
    b. It is associated with a more severe history of alcohol dependence when compared to those with MDD and alcohol dependence
    c. It is longer-lasting than MDD in patients with alcohol dependence
    d. It is associated with a history of independent depressive disorder in first-degree relatives

41. The strongest association between the presence of lifetime AUD and a lifetime anxiety disorder based on literature is seen for:
    a. Obsessive–compulsive disorder (OCD)
    b. Social anxiety disorder
    c. Panic disorder
    d. Generalized anxiety disorder

42. A 28-year-old male presents to your clinic with periodic drinking episodes or binges interspersed with periods of abstinence lasting weeks or months. Based on Emil Jellinek's typology, this would be:
    a. Alpha alcoholism
    b. Beta alcoholism
    c. Delta alcoholism
    d. Epsilon alcoholism

43. A 45-year-old male with a temperament characterized by low novelty seeking and high harm avoidance, late-onset drinking, relatively mild alcohol-related issues and fewer hospitalizations would fit into which of the typologies of AUD:
    a. Cloninger's type II and Babor's type A
    b. Cloninger's type I and Babor's type A
    c. Cloninger's type I and Babor's type B
    d. Cloninger's type II and Babor's type B

44. All of the following are typologies of craving and alcohol dependence proposed by Lesch, *except*:
    a. Craving caused by boredom
    b. Craving caused by stress
    c. Craving caused by mood
    d. Craving caused by compulsion

45. The neurotransmitter imbalance observed in patients with chronic heavy alcohol use, leading to the development of alcohol withdrawal syndrome, is:
    a. Upregulation of GABA and downregulation of glutamate (NMDA receptor) neurotransmission
    b. Downregulation of GABA and upregulation of glutamate (NMDA receptor) neurotransmission
    c. Upregulation of both GABA and glutamate neurotransmission
    d. Downregulation of both GABA and glutamate neurotransmission

46. All of the following are symptoms/signs of alcohol withdrawal, *except*:
    a. Insomnia
    b. Tremors
    c. Yawning
    d. Anxiety

47. All of the following are TRUE about alcohol withdrawal seizures, *except*:
    a. Usually, it begins within 8–24 hours after the patient's last drink and may occur before the blood alcohol level has returned to zero
    b. Generalized tonic–clonic seizures are the most common semiology
    c. Occur singly or in bursts of several seizures over 1–6 hours
    d. Progress to status epilepticus in about 10% of cases

48. All of the following are EEG changes seen in patients with alcohol withdrawal seizures, *except*:
    a. Increased amplitude
    b. Photomyoclonic response
    c. Generalized slowing
    d. Spontaneous paroxysmal activity

49. A 52-year-old male patient with a 25-year history of alcohol dependence presents to the emergency department with a 2-day history of agitation, disorientation, hallucinatory behavior, and tremulousness. The patient's last intake of alcohol was 4 days before the presentation. On examination, the patient has a pulse rate of 120 beats/min, a blood pressure of 150/90 mm Hg, is sweating profusely, and is disoriented in place and person. All of the following are related to this condition, *except*:
    a. Decreased activity of α2 receptors on presynaptic neurons
    b. Increased levels of corticotropin-releasing factor (CRF)

c. Increased activity at the NMDA receptors
d. Increased levels of synaptic magnesium

50. All of the following have been identified as predictors of DT based on recent studies, *except*:
    a. High blood homocysteine and low pyridoxine levels
    b. Low platelet count and low potassium level
    c. Past history of head injury
    d. High magnesium levels

51. The mainstay of treatment for DT is:
    a. Antipsychotic medications
    b. Antiepileptics
    c. Z-drugs
    d. BDZs

52. Long-acting BDZs are preferred over short-acting ones for the treatment of DT because:
    a. Long-acting BDZs have a stronger sedative effect
    b. Short-acting BDZs are more likely to cause addiction
    c. Long-acting BDZs allow for self-tapering and maintain constant serum levels to relieve withdrawal symptoms
    d. Long-acting BDZs have a faster onset of action

53. BDZ refractory delirium, in the context of BDZ treatment for alcohol withdrawal, is defined as:
    a. CIWA-Ar score > 25, and the patient requires ≥200 mg of diazepam in the initial 8 hours
    b. CIWA-Ar score > 25, and the patient requires ≥30 mg of lorazepam in the initial 48 hours
    c. CIWA-Ar score > 25, and the patient requires ≥400 mg of diazepam in the first 8 hours
    d. CIWA-Ar score > 25, and the patient requires ≥45 mg of lorazepam in the initial 48 hours

54. The agents to be considered for the treatment of BDZ refractory delirium are:
    a. Propofol, dexmedetomidine and phenobarbital
    b. Haloperidol, carbamazepine, and valproate
    c. Risperidone and melatonin
    d. Promethazine, trazodone, haloperidol

55. The following statement is TRUE regarding the course of DT:
    a. DT typically starts after 12–24 hours of abrupt cessation of alcohol in a dependent patient, lasts 2–3 days, and resolves spontaneously
    b. DT is a prolonged condition that can last for several weeks

c. DT typically starts after 24–48 hours of abrupt cessation of alcohol in a dependent patient, lasts for 7–10 days, and resolves spontaneously

d. DT typically starts after 48–96 hours of abrupt cessation of alcohol in a dependent patient, lasts 3–4 days and resolves spontaneously within 7 days

56. A 45-year-old male patient with a 20-year history of alcohol dependence presents to the emergency department with a 7-day history of agitation, disorientation, hallucinatory behavior, and tremulousness. The patient's last intake of alcohol was 10 days before the presentation. On examination, the patient has a pulse rate of 84 beats/min, blood pressure of 110/80 mm Hg, diplopia in right lateral gaze, difficulty walking, and impaired recall. The diagnosis is:
    a. Subdural hematoma
    b. Wernicke's encephalopathy
    c. DT
    d. Marchiafava-Bignami syndrome

57. The classic triad of encephalopathy, oculomotor dysfunction, and gait ataxia in Wernicke's encephalopathy is seen in:
    a. 1%
    b. 70%
    c. 16%
    d. 35%

58. The following is NOT TRUE about Wernicke's encephalopathy:
    a. About 80% of patients with Wernicke's encephalopathy who survive develop Korsakoff's syndrome
    b. It is more common in females than in males
    c. Caine's criteria can be used to make a presumptive diagnosis
    d. Variants in the gene *SLC19A2* have been implicated in the pathophysiology

59. All of the following are changes that occur in astrocytes and neurons in a case of Wernicke's encephalopathy, *except*:
    a. Decreased alpha-ketoglutarate dehydrogenase (α-KGDH) activity in astrocytes
    b. Decreased transketolase activity in astrocytes
    c. High intracellular glutamate and low extracellular glutamate
    d. Increased lactate in astrocytes and neurons

60. A relatively specific abnormality for Wernicke's encephalopathy on magnetic resonance imaging (MRI) is:
    a. Mammillary body atrophy
    b. Cortical atrophy
    c. Increased T2 and FLAIR (fluid-attenuated inversion recovery) signals in the red nuclei
    d. Increased T1 signal in medial thalamus

12 Alcohol

61. The acute thiamine supplementation regimen for a suspected case of Wernicke's encephalopathy as operationalized by Caine's criteria is:
    a. 100 mg of oral thiamine thrice a day for 7 days
    b. 500 mg of intramuscular thiamine once a day for 5 days
    c. 500 mg of intravenous thiamine thrice daily for 3–5 days
    d. 100 mg of intravenous thiamine thrice daily for 3–5 days

62. A 52-year-old male patient with alcohol dependence was admitted to the emergency department with an acute onset of fluctuation in consciousness, behavioral disturbances and seizures. On neurological examination, the patient shows increased muscle tone (hypertonia) in his limbs. Imaging shows hyperintense swelling of the corpus callosum on T2-weighted MR sequences. What is the most likely diagnosis based on the patient's symptoms and MRI findings?
    a. Multiple sclerosis (MS)
    b. Wernicke's encephalopathy
    c. Marchiafava–Bignami disease
    d. Cerebral infarction (stroke)

63. The involvement of the central layers with relative sparing of the dorsal and ventral extremes of corpus callosum seen on MRI in Marchiafava–Bignami disease is called:
    a. Hot cross bun sign
    b. Sandwich sign
    c. Burger sign
    d. Taco sign

64. The change observed in the NAA (N-acetyl aspartate)/Cr (creatine) ratio over time in MR spectroscopy of the corpus callosum in Marchiafava–Bignami disease is:
    a. Progressive increase over time
    b. Progressive decrease to a minimum level after the first few months, followed by a partial recovery
    c. Remains constant throughout the disease course
    d. Fluctuates randomly throughout the disease course

65. A 45-year-old man with alcohol dependence for the past 20 years and poor oral intake for the past 6 months presents to the emergency department with a hyperpigmented rash on the dorsum of the hands and feet for the past 1 month, episodes of diarrhea for the past 1 month and features of confusion and reversal of sleep–wake cycle for the past 10 days. The last use of alcohol is 2 days before the presentation. The most likely diagnosis is:
    a. Pellagrous encephalopathy
    b. Dermatitis enteropathica
    c. Psoriatic encephalopathy
    d. Typhoid encephalopathy

66. Alcohol-induced major neurocognitive disorders (persisting dementias) are characterized by:
    a. Global decreases in intellectual functioning, cognitive abilities, and memory are observed, but recent memory difficulties are no more prominent than other elements of this condition
    b. Pronounced anterograde and retrograde amnesia, along with potential impairment in visuospatial, abstract, and other types of learning
    c. A progressive condition characterized by gradual, sequential involvement of multiple cognitive domains
    d. A reversible condition characterized by disproportionate recent memory deficits compared to global cognitive impairment

67. The TRUE statement regarding the pathophysiology of alcohol-induced cerebellar degeneration is:
    a. It mainly affects the granule cells in the cerebellum
    b. Typically occurs with 1–2 years of heavy ethanol use
    c. Midline cerebellar structures, especially the anterior and superior vermis, are predominantly affected
    d. Patient's nutritional status does not increase the risk for its development

68. All of the following are TRUE regarding clinical features, treatment, and course of alcohol-induced cerebellar degeneration, *except*:
    a. Characterized by unsteady gait, impaired standing steadiness, and mild nystagmus
    b. Cerebellar degeneration results from combinations of effects of ethanol, acetaldehyde, and vitamin deficiencies
    c. Treatment requires total abstinence and vitamin supplementation
    d. Complete recovery with total abstinence is seen in a majority of cases

69. "Saturday night palsy" is caused by compression of which among the following:
    a. Ulnar nerve
    b. Radial nerve
    c. Common peroneal nerve
    d. Median nerve

70. The kind of peripheral neuropathy predominantly seen in alcohol-related disease is:
    a. Progressive, predominantly sensory axonal length-dependent neuropathy
    b. Acute, demyelinating polyradiculoneuropathy
    c. Chronic inflammatory demyelinating polyneuropathy (CIDP)
    d. Mononeuropathy multiplex

14 Alcohol

71. The correct statement regarding alcohol-related peripheral neuropathy is:
    a. It has an abrupt onset over days to weeks and almost always affects the upper limbs more than the upper limbs, beginning distally
    b. It has a slow, progressive onset over months to years and almost always affects the lower limbs more than the upper limbs, beginning proximally
    c. It has an abrupt onset over days to weeks and almost always affects the lower limbs more than the upper limbs, beginning proximally
    d. It has a slow, progressive onset over months to years and almost always affects the lower limbs more than the upper limbs, beginning distally

72. Currently, the best validated risk factor for the development of alcohol-related peripheral neuropathy is:
    a. Chronic liver disease
    b. A higher total lifetime dose of ethanol (TLDE)
    c. Smoking
    d. Genetic predisposition

73. The statement that most accurately describes the pattern of muscle involvement in alcohol myopathy is:
    a. Alcohol myopathy affects muscles far from the body's midline (i.e., distal muscles), primarily in the hands and feet symmetrically
    b. Alcohol myopathy most severely affects muscles close to the body's midline (i.e., proximal muscles), primarily the pelvic and shoulder girdles, in a focal and asymmetric fashion
    c. Alcohol myopathy shows a random pattern of muscle involvement with no specific preference for any muscle group
    d. Alcohol myopathy exclusively affects the muscles of the lower extremities bilaterally and symmetrically

74. A 45-year-old alcoholic male complains of muscle weakness and pain. On examination, muscle wasting in the pelvic and shoulder girdles is evident. Additionally, muscle twitching and myotonia are observed. Based on the clinical scenario, what is the most likely diagnosis?
    a. CIDP
    b. Chronic alcoholic myopathy
    c. Guillain–Barré syndrome
    d. Multiple sclerosis

75. Which molecular pathways are increasingly recognized to contribute to alcohol-induced muscle wasting?
    a. Reductions in insulin sensitivity and glucose uptake
    b. Upregulation of pro-inflammatory cytokines

c. Reductions in mammalian target of rapamycin-mediated protein synthesis and excessive protein degradation by activating the lysosomal system
d. Activation of the PI3K-Akt (phosphoinositide-3-kinase–protein kinase B) pathway and increased protein synthesis

76. A 35-year-old man with a history of regular alcohol use presents to the emergency department with a 1-day history of severe headache and two episodes of complex partial seizures. The most likely diagnosis is:
    a. Acute alcohol intoxication
    b. Migraine with aura
    c. Alcohol withdrawal
    d. Cerebral venous thrombosis (CVT)

77. The probable reason why intoxication with alcohol can lead to CVT is:
    a. Alcohol-induced dehydration and hyperviscosity
    b. Alcohol-induced bone marrow suppression
    c. Alcohol-induced sedation and relaxation
    d. Alcohol-induced increase in platelet count

78. All of the following statements regarding alcohol use and acute pancreatitis are TRUE, *except*:
    a. Alcohol use is the most common cause of acute pancreatitis worldwide
    b. The amount of alcohol consumed is the most important risk factor for developing acute pancreatitis
    c. The incidence of acute pancreatitis in patients with alcohol dependence is low (~5/100,000)
    d. The presence of comorbid smoking increases the risk of acute pancreatitis

79. The following statements regarding the pathophysiology of alcohol-associated liver disease are FALSE:
    a. Increased gut-derived endotoxins leading to increased intestinal permeability
    b. Presence of acetaldehyde adducts
    c. Decreased NADH to NAD (nicotinamide adenine dinucleotide) ratio
    d. Increased reactive oxygen species formation

80. The sets of clinical manifestations that are the characteristic signs of alcohol-related liver cirrhosis are:
    a. Gynecomastia, ascites, palmar erythema, jaundice
    b. Anemia, enlargement of parotid and lacrimal glands, rose spots
    c. Hepatosplenomegaly, clubbing, tremors, smiling umbilicus
    d. Spider telangiectasias, enlargement of lacrimal glands, muscle wasting and weakness

16 Alcohol

81. The dose of alcohol consumed over 10–20 years that is associated with the development of severe forms of liver disease, including hepatitis and cirrhosis, is:
    a. 40 g/day
    b. 80 g/day
    c. 120 g/day
    d. 160 g/day

82. The liver biopsy findings that represent abnormal protein aggregate within the hepatocytes and are often observed in individuals with alcohol-related liver disease are:
    a. Steatosis
    b. Ballooning degeneration
    c. Mallory-Denk hyaline bodies
    d. Mallory-Weiss hyaline bodies

83. Increased NADH/NAD ratio due to alcoholism can lead to the following metabolic derangement:
    a. Lactic acidemia, hypoglycemia, hypomagnesemia, hypophosphatemia
    b. Metabolic alkalosis, hypoglycemia, hypomagnesemia, hyperphosphatemia
    c. Lactic acidemia, hypoglycemia, hypermagnesemia, hyperphosphatemia
    d. Metabolic alkalosis, hypoglycemia, hypomagnesemia, hyperphosphatemia

84. The formula to calculate Maddrey's discriminant factor, a prognostic index used in alcoholic hepatitis, is:
    a. 4.6 × [Patient's prothrombin time (PT) in seconds] – (Control PT in seconds) + Serum bilirubin (mg/dL)
    b. 4.6 × (Patient's PT in seconds) + Serum bilirubin (mg/dL)
    c. 4.6 × (Patient's PT in seconds) – (Control PT in seconds) – Serum bilirubin (mg/dL)
    d. 4.6 × (Patient's prothrombin time (PT) in seconds) + (Control PT in seconds) + Serum bilirubin (mg/dL)

85. In alcoholic hepatitis, the AST (aspartate aminotransferase) to ALT (alanine aminotransferase) ratio is often elevated, and commonly their ratio is 2:1 or greater. The main reason for this characteristic ratio in alcoholic hepatitis is:
    a. Alpha-ketoglutarate deficiency
    b. ADH deficiency
    c. Acetaldehyde excess
    d. Pyridoxyl-5-phosphate deficiency

86. A patient with a history of chronic alcohol abuse presents with jaundice, hepatomegaly, and right upper quadrant abdominal pain. These clinical symptoms are suggestive of the following:
    a. Alcoholic hepatitis
    b. Alcoholic cirrhosis
    c. Alcoholic fatty liver disease
    d. Acute pancreatitis

87. The type of alcohol-related liver disease that is completely reversible if the individual abstains from alcohol consumption is:
    a. Alcoholic hepatitis
    b. Alcoholic fatty liver disease
    c. Alcoholic cirrhosis
    d. Alcoholic liver failure

88. The acute effects of alcohol on the circulatory system in adults include all of the following, *except*:
    a. Increased heart rate
    b. Increased blood pressure
    c. Increased cardiac output
    d. Increased ejection fraction

89. The most likely mechanism by which alcohol use may lead to cardiomyopathy is:
    a. Alcohol inhibits the production of red blood cells, leading to reduced oxygen supply to the heart
    b. Alcohol increases cholesterol levels, leading to plaque formation in coronary arteries
    c. At high doses, alcohol acts as a striated-muscle toxin, deteriorating the heart muscle
    d. Alcohol induces abnormal electrical signals in the heart, leading to arrhythmias

90. The term "holiday heart" refers to:
    a. Ischemic heart disease caused by excessive alcohol consumption
    b. An acute cardiac rhythm disturbance related to heavy ethanol consumption in a person without other clinical evidence of heart disease
    c. A psychological disorder related to holiday celebrations and alcohol consumption
    d. Mitral valve prolapse caused by excessive alcohol consumption

91. The mechanisms by which alcohol use leads to increased blood pressure include all of the following, *except*:
    a. Increased sympathetic drive
    b. Decreased levels of corticotropin-releasing hormone (CRH)
    c. Impaired baroreceptor reflex
    d. Worsening of sleep apnea

92. All of the following are commonly observed electrolyte disturbances in patients with AUD, *except*:
    a. Hypokalemia
    b. Hypophosphatemia
    c. Hypermagnesemia
    d. Hypocalcemia

18 Alcohol

93. All of the following are TRUE about the effects of alcohol on lipogenesis, *except*:
    a. Increases triglyceride synthesis
    b. Increases high-density lipoprotein (HDL) fraction of cholesterol
    c. Increases NADH/NAD ratio
    d. Increases low-density lipoprotein fraction of cholesterol

94. The following is TRUE regarding the effects of alcohol on the hematopoietic system:
    a. Decreases the production of white blood cells and impairs the ability of those cells to migrate to sites of infection; affects the stem cells that produce the red blood components, increasing the average size of red cells
    b. Increases the production of white blood cells but impairs the ability of those cells to migrate to sites of infection; affects the stem cells that produce the red blood components, increasing the average size of red cells
    c. Decreases the production of white blood cells and impairs the ability of those cells to migrate to sites of infection; increases the production of red blood cell components at the bone marrow level
    d. Decreases the production of white blood cells; increases the production of red blood cells and platelets

95. The following is TRUE about alcohol use and cancers:
    a. It probably reflects alcohol-related immune system suppression and the direct effects of ethanol and acetaldehyde on mucosal membranes
    b. Heightened rates of malignant tumors in patients with alcohol use become insignificant when the impact of smoking and poor nutrition is considered
    c. Acetaldehyde helps in lysis of tumor cells
    d. Cancer is the most common cause of premature death in individuals with AUDs

96. The elevated risk of breast cancer in women with AUDs is due to:
    a. Increased levels of estradiol
    b. Increased levels of progesterone
    c. Increased levels of testosterone
    d. Increased levels of prolactin

97. The potential consequences of chronic alcohol use on sexual functioning in men include all, *except*:
    a. Decreased libido
    b. Premature ejaculation

c. Decreased sexual desire
d. Decreased risk-taking behavior leading to reduced sexual activity

98. The potential sexual issues that may arise in women with chronic alcohol use include all, *except*:
    a. Decreased desire
    b. Decreased vaginal lubrication
    c. Difficulty in achieving orgasm
    d. Dyspareunia

99. In individuals without AUD, the following is TRUE regarding the effect of alcohol on sleep:
    a. In the latter half of the sleep period, it promotes deep sleep
    b. In the latter half of the sleep period, it increases rapid eye movement (REM) sleep
    c. In the initial half of the sleep period, it increases REM sleep
    d. In the initial half of the sleep period, it leads to increased sleep latency

100. In individuals with AUD, all of the following is TRUE regarding the effect of alcohol on sleep, *except*:
    a. Decreased sleep latency
    b. Decreased REM sleep
    c. Decreased total sleep time
    d. Decreased stage 4 sleep

101. Which among these is not an Food and Drug Administration (FDA)-approved agent for the treatment of AUD?
    a. Acamprosate
    b. Disulfiram
    c. Naltrexone
    d. Baclofen

102. The following best describes the mechanism of action of disulfiram in the treatment of AUD:
    a. Disulfiram inhibits the enzyme ADH, leading to the accumulation of acetaldehyde
    b. Disulfiram irreversibly inhibits the enzyme ALDH, leading to the accumulation of acetaldehyde
    c. Disulfiram inhibits the enzyme ALDH reversibly, leading to the accumulation of acetaldehyde
    d. Disulfiram blocks the effects of alcohol on the GABA receptors, reducing alcohol's pleasurable effects

103. The metabolite of disulfiram, which chelates copper ions, thereby inhibiting dopamine beta-hydroxylase activity, leading to psychosis, is:
    a. Diethyldithiocarbamate (DDC)
    b. Methyl isocyanate (MIC)
    c. Dichlorodiphenyltrichloroethane (DDT)
    d. Hydrogen sulfide

104. The potential candidates to start disulfiram for the treatment of AUD are:
    a. Patients who are motivated for treatment, want total abstinence, can receive supervised dosing, and can understand disulfiram-ethanol reaction (DER)
    b. Patients with a history of cocaine dependence, irrespective of their motivation for treatment and abstinence goals
    c. Patients who are noncompliant with other AUD treatments need alternative therapy
    d. Patients who are not motivated for treatment but severe dysfunction is present, and family members want to give some medication for the patient's abstinence

105. The mechanism by which ascorbic acid (vitamin C) can assist in reducing the duration and severity of disulfiram-induced psychosis is:
    a. It acts as a dopamine antagonist, blocking psychotic symptoms
    b. It inhibits the metabolism of disulfiram, reducing its concentration in the body
    c. It increases the Ph of the urine, promoting the excretion of disulfiram from the body
    d. It increases the urine's acidity (lowers the Ph), promoting the excretion of disulfiram and its metabolites

106. The statement that most accurately describes acute liver injury due to disulfiram (tetraethyl thiuram disulfide) is:
    a. Acute liver injury due to disulfiram is a common adverse effect observed at higher doses and in patients with underlying liver disease
    b. The risk of acute liver injury from disulfiram is dose-related and primarily affects patients with preexisting liver conditions
    c. This risk seems unrelated to an underlying liver disease, is not dose-related, and is thought to result from a hypersensitivity reaction involving P450 cytochrome enzymes
    d. Acute liver injury due to disulfiram is primarily observed in patients with AUD and chronic alcohol consumption

107. The Danish researchers responsible for the serendipitous discovery of disulfiram's effects on alcohol dependence are:
    a. Jens Christian Skou and Henning von Tresckow
    b. Hans von Euler-Chelpin and Arthur Harden
    c. Erik Jacobsen and Jens Hald
    d. Henrik Dam and Edward Doisy

108. DER can manifest with various symptoms, such as flushing, tachycardia, hypotension, and confusion. These symptoms result from:
    a. An allergic reaction to disulfiram
    b. Increased dopamine levels in the brain
    c. Accumulation of acetaldehyde upon alcohol consumption
    d. Direct neurotoxic effects of disulfiram

109. The combination of medications that may potentially lead to a DER are:
    a. Fluoxetine, cetirizine, and metronidazole
    b. Amlodipine, aspirin, and lorazepam
    c. Levothyroxine, ibuprofen, and omeprazole
    d. Sertraline, diphenhydramine, and cephalexin

110. The most appropriate timing to initiate disulfiram therapy after the last use of alcohol is:
    a. Immediately after the last alcoholic drink
    b. 6 hours after the last alcoholic drink
    c. 72 hours after the last alcoholic drink
    d. 24 hours after the last alcoholic drink

111. The half-life of the active metabolite of disulfiram-diethyldithiocarbamic acid methyl ester in the treatment of AUD is:
    a. 24–48 hours
    b. 6–12 hours
    c. 72–96 hours
    d. 1 week

112. The proposed mechanism by which naltrexone helps to reduce alcohol consumption in humans is:
    a. Increasing the release of dopamine in the brain to reduce alcohol cravings
    b. Blocking opioid receptors in the brain, reducing alcohol's pleasurable effects
    c. Enhancing the metabolism of alcohol to acetaldehyde, reducing its intoxicating effects
    d. Stimulating the production of endorphins decreases alcohol dependence

113. The approximate plasma half-life of naltrexone, when administered orally, is:
    a. 6–8 hours
    b. 10–12 hours
    c. 14–19 hours
    d. 24–48 hours

114. The COMBINE trial was a landmark clinical trial evaluating the efficacy of different medications and behavioral therapies in treating

22 Alcohol

alcohol dependence. The TRUE statement about the results of the COMBINE trial is:
a. Naltrexone combined with disulfiram was the most effective treatment for alcohol dependence
b. Acamprosate was significantly more effective than other medications in reducing alcohol cravings
c. A combination of naltrexone and cognitive behavioral therapy (CBT) was superior to either treatment alone
d. Combining acamprosate and CBT was superior to either treatment alone

115. In the treatment of AUD, the outcome for which naltrexone demonstrates the best efficacy is:
a. Achieving complete abstinence from alcohol
b. Reducing alcohol cravings and withdrawal symptoms
c. Preventing return to heavy drinking and reducing percent drinking days
d. Improving social functioning and interpersonal relationships

116. In patients receiving naltrexone for the treatment of AUD, the recommended frequency of liver function test (LFT) monitoring, according to the American Society of Addiction Medicine (ASAM) guidelines, is:
a. Baseline LFTs and monitoring at 6 months and 1 year
b. Baseline LFTs and monitoring at 3 months and 6 months
c. Baseline LFTs and monitoring at 1 month, 3 months, and then periodically afterward
d. Baseline LFTs only; no further monitoring required

117. The current status of research on the predictive utility of the Asn40Asp polymorphism of the μ-opioid receptor (*OPRM1*) gene in response to naltrexone treatment is as follows:
a. Studies consistently demonstrate a stronger effect of naltrexone in Asp40 carriers
b. Studies consistently show no effect of the Asn40Asp polymorphism on naltrexone response
c. The predictive utility of the Asn40Asp polymorphism in naltrexone response is well established
d. Research findings are mixed; some studies show a stronger effect in Asp40 carriers, while others do not

118. Naltrexone, either alone or in combination, has FDA approval for all of the conditions, *except*:
a. Opioid dependence
b. Obesity
c. Alcohol dependence
d. Nicotine dependence

119. In patients with a history of hepatitis or liver disease, the precaution that should be taken before starting naltrexone treatment for alcohol dependence is:
    a. Frequent alcohol consumption to gauge the severity of dependence
    b. A liver biopsy to assess the degree of liver damage
    c. Consultation with a psychiatrist to evaluate mental health status
    d. A thorough medical history and liver function tests

120. The profile of patients with alcohol dependence for whom naltrexone treatment may be best suited is as follows:
    a. Early onset, positive family history, impulsive traits; the goal is harm reduction
    b. Early onset, negative family history, impulsive traits; the goal is complete abstinence
    c. Late-onset, positive family history, impulsive traits, the goal is harm reduction
    d. Late-onset, negative family history of alcoholism, impulsive traits; the goal is complete abstinence

121. The recommended dosing schedule for long-acting injectable naltrexone (extended-release naltrexone) is as follows:
    a. 380-mg deep intramuscular dose once every week
    b. 380-mg deep intramuscular dose once every 2 weeks
    c. 380-mg deep intramuscular dose once every 3 weeks
    d. 380-mg deep intramuscular dose once every 4 weeks

122. An absolute contraindication for the use of injectable preparation of naltrexone is:
    a. Patients who have previously exhibited hypersensitivity to naltrexone, polylactide-co-glycolide (PLG), carboxymethylcellulose, or any other diluent components
    b. Obesity
    c. Need for opioid analgesics within the next 30 days
    d. All of the above

123. The characteristic pharmacokinetics of extended-release injectable naltrexone is:
    a. It exhibits a single peak plasma concentration after injection
    b. The drug reaches its peak plasma concentration within a few hours after injection
    c. It shows biphasic release with two distinct peaks of plasma concentration
    d. The drug has a short half-life, requiring frequent dosing

Alcohol

124. The possible side effects of extended-release injectable naltrexone include:
    a. Allergic reactions, skin rash, and hives
    b. Headache and insomnia
    c. Gastrointestinal side effects, injection site reactions, muscle cramps, and dizziness
    d. Increased appetite and weight gain

125. The TRUE statement when comparing the oral and injectable forms of naltrexone is:
    a. The oral form is more effective in achieving abstinence than the injectable form
    b. Both forms have similar rates of treatment adherence and periods of abstinence
    c. The oral form is associated with higher rates of treatment adherence and longer periods of abstinence than the injectable form
    d. The injectable form is associated with higher rates of treatment adherence and longer periods of abstinence than the oral form

126. The approximate half-life of acamprosate is:
    a. 12–50 hours
    b. 6–8 hours
    c. 12–16 hours
    d. 20–33 hours

127. The oral bioavailability of acamprosate is:
    a. 2–11 %
    b. 30–40%
    c. 50–60%
    d. 80–90%

128. Acamprosate has been noted to have structural similarities to all of the following amino acids, *except*:
    a. Glutamate
    b. Tyrosine
    c. Aspartate
    d. Taurine

129. The possible mechanism through which acamprosate exerts its therapeutic effect in the treatment of alcohol dependence is:
    a. Acamprosate acts as a CNS stimulant, increasing alertness and reducing alcohol cravings
    b. Acamprosate enhances the effects of alcohol, leading to reduced consumption and dependence
    c. Acamprosate increases dopamine release in the brain, promoting a sense of reward and reducing alcohol cravings
    d. Acamprosate modulates the GABA and glutamatergic neurotransmission, reducing excitatory signals and reducing alcohol cravings and relapse

130. The following statements are TRUE regarding the pharmacokinetics of acamprosate:
    a. Acamprosate has a long half-life and has good oral bioavailability
    b. The liver primarily metabolizes it, leading to potential drug–drug interactions
    c. The drug reaches peak plasma concentrations rapidly after oral administration
    d. Acamprosate is eliminated unchanged in the urine

131. The following are the most commonly reported side effects of acamprosate:
    a. Nausea, pruritis and diarrhea
    b. Sedation and drowsiness
    c. Increased heart rate and palpitations
    d. Muscle pain and weakness

132. The patients for whom acamprosate may be most beneficial are:
    a. Patients who drink for rewarding effects and to get high
    b. Patients who want to reduce their alcohol intake but do not want complete abstinence
    c. Patients who are experiencing acute alcohol withdrawal symptoms
    d. Patients who want complete abstinence from alcohol

133. For individuals with a weight of >60 kg, the daily dosage of acamprosate is:
    a. 666 mg in the morning and 666 mg in the evening
    b. 1,332 mg in the morning
    c. 333 mg in the morning and 999 mg in the evening
    d. 666 mg in the morning, afternoon, and evening

134. The typical duration of acamprosate treatment for alcohol dependence in individuals weighing >60 kg is:
    a. 1 week
    b. 1 month
    c. 3 months
    d. 6 months

135. In the book "Le Dernier Verre", the scientist and author of the book who relates how he cured himself with a high dose of baclofen, is:
    a. Olivier Amiesen
    b. Jacques Monod
    c. Luc Montagnier
    d. Jonas Salk

136. The follow-up analysis from the BACLAD group revealed that in subjects with alcoholic liver disease, baclofen administration resulted in which of the following findings?
    a. Increased time to relapse and decreased percentage of days abstinent

b. Decreased time to lapse and increased percentage of days abstinent
c. Increased time to lapse and increased percentage of days abstinent
d. Decreased time to relapse and decreased percentage of days abstinent

137. The approximate half-life of baclofen is:
    a. 1–2 hours
    b. 4–6 hours
    c. 812 hours
    d. 24–36 hours

138. Regarding the pharmacokinetics and excretion of baclofen, the correct statement is:
    a. Baclofen is metabolized in the liver and excreted through the kidneys unchanged
    b. Baclofen is primarily metabolized in the kidneys and excreted through the liver unchanged
    c. Baclofen is primarily metabolized in the liver and excreted through the bile
    d. Baclofen is mainly metabolized in the kidneys and excreted through the urine

139. Baclofen intoxication can lead to serious consequences and life-threatening situations. The symptoms that are commonly observed in individuals experiencing baclofen intoxication are:
    a. Increased muscle rigidity, respiratory depression
    b. Hyperthermia and severe dehydration
    c. Nausea, vomiting, and diarrhea
    d. Hypotonia, dizziness, and seizures

140. What are the common side effects of using baclofen, a medication for muscle spasticity and AUD?
    a. Increased appetite, weight gain
    b. Excessive sweating, fever
    c. Nausea, vomiting, diarrhea
    d. Drowsiness, dizziness, urinary retention

141. The primary mechanism of action of baclofen is:
    a. Stimulation of $GABA_A$ receptors
    b. Stimulation of $GABA_B$ receptors
    c. Inhibition of serotonin receptors
    d. Activation of NMDA receptors

142. Of the anti-craving agents for alcohol dependence mentioned below, the safest option for individuals with coexisting end-stage alcohol-related liver disease is:
    a. Naltrexone
    b. Baclofen
    c. Ondansetron
    d. Disulfiram

143. The primary mechanism of action of gabapentin, a medication commonly used to treat epilepsy, neuropathic pain, and other conditions, is:
    a. Inhibition of serotonin reuptake
    b. Activation of GABAergic receptors
    c. Blockade of alpha 2d subunit of voltage-gated calcium channels
    d. Antagonism of NMDA receptors

144. Gabapentin is primarily metabolized through:
    a. Hepatic metabolism
    b. Renal metabolism
    c. Hepatobiliary metabolism
    d. Gastrointestinal metabolism

145. The adverse effects that should be taken into consideration while prescribing gabapentin, especially when combined with other medications, are:
    a. Nausea and vomiting
    b. Hypertension and tachycardia
    c. Respiratory depression
    d. Dry mouth and constipation

146. The typical dosage range of gabapentin, when used as an anti-craving medication in the treatment of AUD, is:
    a. 100–300 mg/day
    b. 500–1,000 mg/day
    c. 1,500–3,000 mg/day
    d. 4,000–6,000 mg/day

147. The following are common side effects associated with the use of topiramate, a medication used to treat epilepsy, migraines, and AUD:
    a. Dizziness, dry mouth, and constipation
    b. Decreased appetite, blurred vision, and memory problems
    c. Fatigue, nausea, and increased appetite
    d. Headache, insomnia, and muscle pain

148. A single nucleotide polymorphism (rs2832407) in GRIK1, encoding the kainate GluK1 receptor subunit, was found to mediate substance use outcomes about:
    a. Acamprosate
    b. Topiramate
    c. Lamotrigine
    d. Baclofen

149. The μ- and κ-opioid receptor antagonist that has received approval from the European Medicines Agency in 2013 for treatment of alcohol dependence is:
    a. Naltrexone
    b. Nalbuphine
    c. Nalmefene
    d. Naloxone

150. In patients with AUD, polymorphisms in the genes coding for serotonin 5-HT3 receptor subtypes were found to predict response to treatment with:
    a. Topiramate
    b. Aripiprazole
    c. Ondansetron
    d. Fluoxetine

151. In patients with comorbid depression and AUD, a large randomized controlled trial (RCT) found evidence for improvement in depressive symptoms and alcohol use for a combination of naltrexone with:
    a. Fluoxetine
    b. Escitalopram
    c. Desvenlafaxine
    d. Sertraline

152. Alcoholics Anonymous was started by:
    a. Bob Smith and Bill Wilson
    b. Alan Marlatt and John Gordon
    c. William Miller and Stephen Rollnick
    d. James Prochaska and Carlo Di Clemente

153. Al-Anon is a self-help group for:
    a. Men with alcohol dependence
    b. Teenagers with alcohol dependence
    c. Women with alcohol dependence
    d. Friends and relatives of those with alcohol dependence

154. Project MATCH compared all of the following treatments for alcohol-abusing or dependent patients, *except*:
    a. Motivation enhancement therapy
    b. Contingency management
    c. Cognitive behavioral therapy
    d. 12-Step facilitation therapy

155. The following is usually a primary requirement in most transplant programs to consider a patient with alcohol-related chronic liver disease for a liver transplant:
    a. Demonstrating the ability to quit alcohol cold turkey
    b. Being a nonsmoker
    c. Completing a detoxification program
    d. Maintaining sobriety for a specific duration (e.g., 6 months)

156. The TRUE statement regarding liver transplantation for alcoholic liver disease is:
    a. It should not be considered for patients with acute severe alcoholic hepatitis
    b. Alcohol-related liver disease is the leading indication for liver transplantation worldwide

c. Patients with alcoholic liver disease have worse transplant outcomes than other liver disease etiologies
   d. Liver transplantation is not an effective treatment for alcoholic liver disease

157. The success of liver transplantation in patients with alcoholic liver disease heavily relies on the following:
   a. The availability of highly specialized surgical teams
   b. The patient's age at the time of transplantation
   c. The patient's motivation and commitment to long-term sobriety
   d. The frequency of alcohol consumption before transplantation

158. The phenomenon known as "telescoping", described in the context of substance use disorders (SUDs) amongst women, is:
   a. The accelerated progression from substance dependence to abstinence
   b. The phenomenon of substance users entering treatment at an older age
   c. The slower progression from substance use initiation to the development of SUDs
   d. The accelerated progression from the initiation of substance use to the development of SUDs and entry into treatment

159. Women appear to be at greater risk of developing ALD for a given level of alcohol consumption than men because:
   a. Lower gastric ADH activity
   b. Lower hepatic alcohol metabolic rate
   c. Lower fat-to-water ratio
   d. Lower liver mass per kilogram of body weight

160. All of the following are screening instruments validated for alcohol use in pregnancy, *except*:
   a. CAGE
   b. T-ACE
   c. TWEAK
   d. AUDIT-C

161. All of the following are signs of fetal alcohol syndrome, *except*:
   a. Prominent upper lip
   b. Absent philtrum
   c. Flat nasal bridge
   d. Syndactyly

162. A 28-year-old laborer presents with vomiting, headache, confusion, and diminution of vision, which started 1–2 hours after consumption of alcohol from a local liquor shop. On clarification, it was found that his friends who had consumed alcohol with him also had the same symptoms. The most likely diagnosis is:
   a. DER
   b. Methanol poisoning
   c. Acute glaucoma
   d. Giant cell arteritis

163. The preferred drug for the treatment of methanol poisoning is:
    a. Fomepizole
    b. Ethanol
    c. BDZs
    d. Cyclopyrrolones

164. The following statement is TRUE about AUD in the older adults:
    a. Alcohol withdrawal may be less severe and less prolonged in older patients than in younger ones
    b. Shorter-acting BDZs are preferred in older patients to reduce the effect of accumulation and decrease the risk of falls
    c. Disulfiram has the best evidence for treatment in older adults
    d. The front-loading approach should be preferred over the symptom-triggered approach to manage alcohol withdrawal in older patients

165. The legally acceptable limit for blood alcohol levels while driving in India is:
    a. <30 mg/100 mL of blood
    b. <20 mg/100 mL of blood
    c. <80 mg/100 mL of blood
    d. <120 mg/100 mL of blood

166. The states in India where the prohibition of alcohol is currently in force are:
    a. Bihar, Gujarat, Jammu and Kashmir
    b. Mizoram, Gujarat, Nagaland
    c. Bengal, Bihar, Gujarat
    d. Andaman and Nicobar, Bihar, Gujarat

167. All of the following Indian states have prohibited alcohol at some point after independence, *except*:
    a. Haryana
    b. Tamil Nadu
    c. Andhra Pradesh
    d. Madhya Pradesh

168. In the Indian Motor Vehicles Act, drunk driving comes under:
    a. Section 185
    b. Section 186
    c. Section 189
    d. Section 195

169. Mr X, following a road traffic accident, was bedridden for 3 days, following which he goes into DT and is brought to hospital. During this time, he misrecognizes and stabs his wife, resulting in her death. The section applicable in this case is:
    a. Section 85 IPC
    b. Section 84 IPC
    c. Section 201 IPC
    d. Section 94 IPC

170. Mr Z and his friend, on a weekend, go to a party, consume alcohol and engage in sexual intercourse following alcohol use. Subsequently, his friend filed a complaint that Mr Z had raped her. The section applicable in this case is:
    a. Section 89 IPC
    b. Section 90 IPC
    c. Section 94 IPC
    d. Section 102 IPC

TRUE OR FALSE

171. Due to the high surface area, ethanol absorption occurs more rapidly from the stomach than from the small intestine.
172. Ethanol metabolism proceeds via zero-order kinetics at BECs > 10 mg% and by first-order kinetics at BECs < 10 mg%.
173. CYP2E1 is inhibited by chronic ethanol consumption, resulting in decreased clearance of its substrates.
174. Alcohol does not bind as a direct agonist at receptors in the brain but rather appears to be sequestered in transmembrane water pockets and modulates receptors (termed ethanol-receptive elements).
175. Alcohol increases the release of certain opioid peptides (such as dynorphin) from rat pituitary glands.
176. Alcohol has been shown to inhibit the function of a nucleoside transporter, leading to increased extracellular adenosine levels.
177. Heteromeric nicotinic receptors composed of $\alpha\beta$ subunits appear to be potentiated by ethanol, whereas homomeric receptors composed of just α subunits are inhibited by ethanol.
178. In animal studies, cannabinoid 1 (CB1) antagonists such as rimonabant reduce ethanol preference in wild-type mice.
179. The definition of one standard drink/unit as per World Health Organization (WHO) given in AUDIT is one standard drink/unit is equal to 14 g of absolute alcohol.
180. The presence of attention-deficit/hyperactivity disorder (ADHD) is not associated with an earlier onset of alcohol use.
181. The presence of comorbid alcohol use is a contraindication for prescribing stimulants to treat comorbid ADHD.
182. A strong association has been found between the genetic polymorphism (rs738409) of patatin-like phospholipase domain-containing protein 3 (PNPLA3) and the progression of ALD.
183. The specificity of transient elastography for detecting fibrosis in patients with ALD is somewhat lower than reported for other etiologies, such as viral hepatitis.
184. Sialosis, a painless symmetrical enlargement of the parotid glands, is common in the context of AUD.
185. Acute alcohol ingestion leads to lower esophageal sphincter (LES) contraction.
186. Patients with AUD appear to be at an increased risk of developing obstructive sleep apnea.

187. The incidence of gynecomastia increases in alcoholic cirrhosis, primarily because of increased levels of androstenedione, a precursor for estrogen synthesis.
188. Nightmares and vivid dreams seen in alcohol withdrawal reflect an REM rebound phenomenon.
189. Alcohol inhibits oxytocin release and reduces milk production in lactating mothers.
190. Women get more intoxicated with the same doses of alcohol than men due to higher total body water content, leading to higher BACs and higher concentrations of gastric ADH.
191. Women with addiction have higher rates of anxiety, depression, eating disorders, and emotionally unstable personality disorder, while men with addiction have higher rates of antisocial personality disorder and ADHD.
192. Alcohol use is globally the most common cause of fatal and non-fatal road traffic accidents.
193. As per the Global Burden of Disease Study, alcohol use was the third leading risk factor for deaths and DALYs (disability-adjusted life years) in 2016.

FILL IN THE BLANKS

194. The phenomenon of acute functional tolerance, where behavioral impairment and subjective feelings of intoxication related to alcohol are much greater at a given BEC when the concentrations are ascending rather than descending, is termed _____.
195. The phenomenon where a person with alcohol dependence requires a higher dose of other depressants, such as BDZs, for sleep induction is called _____.
196. An increase in the pharmacological and physiological response to alcohol after repeated exposures is termed _____.
197. Animal studies have demonstrated that submitting animals to repeated alcohol withdrawal episodes increases their risk of withdrawal seizures. This is termed _____.
198. Legal and regulatory changes in the legal alcohol environment, which reduce or eliminate regulatory control over aspects of availability, cost, and outlet locations, typically resulting in increased consumption and related consequences, are called _____.
199. According to the National Mental Health Survey, 2016, the treatment gap for AUD is _____.

Alcohol

200. The FDA-approved drug for smoking cessation with evidence of efficacy in double-blind RCTs for the treatment of alcohol dependence is _____.

201. _____ is linked to excessive alcohol use and is characterized by massive bleeding caused by tears in the mucosa at the cardioesophageal junction after vomiting.

202. _____ is a condition for further study in DSM-5 to encompass the full range of developmental disabilities associated with exposure to alcohol in utero.

203. The sections of IPC (Indian Penal Code) that deal with criminal responsibility of an intoxicated person are _____

■ MATCH THE FOLLOWING

204. Match the medications with their FDA-approved doses.

A. Acamprosate	a. 50 mg/day
B. Naltrexone	b. 250 mg/day
C. Disulfiram	c. 1,998 mg/day

205. Match the signs of Wernicke's encephalopathy with the time course of resolution with thiamine treatment.

A. Oculomotor abnormalities	a. Within weeks
B. Gait ataxia	b. Within hours
C. Encephalopathy	c. Within days

■ ANSWER KEY

1. c	2. d	3. c	4. c	5. c	6. a	7. d	8. c
9. a	10. c	11. b	12. a	13. a	14. c	15. d	16. c
17. c	18. a	19. b	20. a	21. d	22. a	23. d	24. b
25. d	26. d	27. c	28. b	29. c	30. c	31. a	32. c
33. a	34. d	35. b	36. a	37. a	38. d	39. b	40. b
41. c	42. d	43. b	44. a	45. b	46. c	47. d	48. c
49. d	50. d	51. d	52. c	53. c	54. a	55. d	56. b
57. c	58. b	59. c	60. a	61. c	62. c	63. b	64. b
65. a	66. a	67. c	68. d	69. b	70. a	71. d	72. b
73. b	74. b	75. c	76. d	77. a	78. a	79. c	80. a
81. d	82. c	83. a	84. a	85. d	86. a	87. b	88. d
89. c	90. b	91. b	92. c	93. c	94. a	95. a	96. a
97. d	98. d	99. b	100. a	101. d	102. b	103. a	104. a
105. d	106. c	107. c	108. c	109. a	110. d	111. b	112. b

113. b	114. c	115. c	116. c	117. d	118. d	119. d	120. a
121. d	122. a	123. c	124. c	125. d	126. d	127. a	128. b
129. d	130. d	131. a	132. d	133. d	134. d	135. a	136. c
137. b	138. d	139. d	140. d	141. b	142. b	143. c	144. b
145. c	146. c	147. b	148. b	149. c	150. c	151. d	152. a
153. d	154. b	155. d	156. b	157. c	158. d	159. a	160. a
161. a	162. b	163. a	164. b	165. a	166. b	167. d	168. a
169. b	170. b						

TRUE OR FALSE

171. False	172. True	173. False	174. True
175. False	176. True	177. True	178. True
179. False	180. False	181. False	182. True
183. True	184. True	185. False	186. True
187. True	188. True	189. True	190. False
191. True	192. True	193. False	

FILL IN THE BLANKS

194. Mellanby effect	195. Cross tolerance	196. Sensitization
197. Kindling	198. Deregulation	199. 86.3%
200. Varenicline	201. Mallory–Weiss syndrome	202. Neurobehavioral Disorder Associated with Prenatal Alcohol Exposure (ND-PAE)
203. Sections 85 and 86		

MATCH THE FOLLOWING

204. A—c.	B—a.	C—b.
205. A—b.	B—c.	C—a.

FURTHER READING

1. El-Guebaly N, Carrà G, Galanter M, Baldacchino AM, editors. Textbook of Addiction Treatment: International Perspectives. Switzerland: Springer International Publishing; 2021.
2. Miller PM. Principles of Addiction: Comprehensive Addictive Behaviors and Disorders, volumes 1 to 3. San Diego: Academic Press; 2013.
3. Miller S. The ASAM Principles of Addiction Medicine, 6th edition. Philadelphia: Lippincott Williams & Wilkins; 2018.
4. Sadock BJ, Sadock VA, Ruiz P. Kaplan & Sadock's Comprehensive Textbook of Psychiatry, 10th edition. Philadelphia: Lippincott Williams & Wilkins; 2017.

CHAPTER 2

Nicotine

Preethy Kathiresan, Ankita Chattopadhyay, Tanmay Joshi

1. Which of the following is a serious/severe side effect of bupropion?
   a. Increased sedation
   b. Seizures
   c. Nausea
   d. Insomnia

2. What is the mechanism of action of varenicline?
   a. Partial agonist at α4β2 receptors
   b. Antagonist at α4β2 receptors
   c. Partial agonist at α2β4 receptors
   d. Antagonist at α2β4 receptors

3. What does 5As stand for in Brief Intervention for Tobacco?
   a. Ask, Assess, Advise, Avoid, Assist
   b. Ask, Advice, Assist, Arrange, Avoid
   c. Ask, Assess, Advise, Avoid, Assist
   d. Ask, Assess, Advise, Assist, Arrange

4. A 23-year-old male reports smoking around 10 cigarettes daily for the past 5 years. He wants to quit cigarettes but reports a significant craving for the same. The treating doctor prescribes him bupropion. What is the dose of bupropion that has to be prescribed for this person?
   a. 300 mg for the first week, followed by a decrease in dose to 150 mg
   b. 150 mg for the first week, followed by an increase in dose to 300 mg
   c. 10 mg for the first week, followed by an increase in dose to 20 mg
   d. 20 mg for the first week, followed by a decrease in dose to 10 mg

5. Which is the most common form of smokeless tobacco use in India?
   a. Gutkha
   b. Khaini
   c. Zarda
   d. Gul

6. Which of these medications is not used in the management of nicotine addiction?
   a. Buprenorphine
   b. Bupropion
   c. Varenicline
   d. Nortriptyline

7. The psychoactive effect of nicotine on the central nervous system is:
   a. Stimulant
   b. Depressant
   c. Hallucinogen
   d. Dissociation

8. A 23-year-old male felt an increased alertness and ability to focus on studies after taking nicotine for the first time. Which receptor is responsible for this mentally alerting action of nicotine?
   a. α4β2 receptor
   b. α2β4 receptor
   c. α7 receptor
   d. None of the above

9. Which of the following is not included in the treatment of tobacco dependence in treatment guidelines by the National Tobacco Control Programme (NTCP) India?
   a. Nicotine replacement therapy (NRT)
   b. Bupropion
   c. Nortriptyline
   d. Varenicline

10. MPOWER is a policy package intended to assist in the country-level implementation of effective interventions to reduce the demand for tobacco, as ratified by the World Health Organization (WHO) Framework Convention on Tobacco Control. MPOWER is an acronym for MPOWER measures, which includes all of the following, *except*:
    a. M—Monitor tobacco use and prevention policies
    b. P—Protect people from tobacco use
    c. O—Offer help to prevent tobacco use
    d. W—Warn about the dangers of tobacco

11. What is the primary cause of EVALI (e-cigarette- or vaping-associated lung injury)?
    a. Vitamin E
    b. Nicotine
    c. Vitamin A
    d. Carbon monoxide (CO)

12. According to the Global Adult Tobacco Survey 2 (GATS 2) 2016–2017, overall tobacco use declined by:
    a. 16%
    b. 8%
    c. 4%
    d. 6%

13. Which factors can contribute to individual differences in nicotine metabolism and subsequent smoking behavior?
    a. Socioeconomic status
    b. Genetic variations in *CYP2A6*
    c. Age of smoking initiation
    d. Frequency of exposure to secondhand smoke

14. Which of the following is not a part of the 5Rs in enhancing motivation to quit tobacco?
    a. Relevance
    b. Resistance
    c. Risks
    d. Repetition

15. What is the primary route of nicotine absorption in smokers?
    a. Pulmonary absorption
    b. Oral absorption
    c. Dermal absorption
    d. Nasal absorption
16. Bupropion acts by blocking which of the following transporters?
    a. Norepinephrine and dopamine reuptake transporters
    b. Dopamine and GABA (gamma-aminobutyric acid) reuptake transporters
    c. Norepinephrine and GABA reuptake transporters
    d. GABA and serotonin reuptake transporters
17. The World No Tobacco Day is celebrated on:
    a. May 31
    b. September 10
    c. October 10
    d. June 31
18. A 38-year-old male was referred by his physician for his regular nicotine-containing cigarette intake. Upon interviewing him, which variable would be the strongest predictor of nicotine addiction?
    a. The time to first cigarette and the total number of nicotine-containing cigarettes daily
    b. The presence of a respiratory or cardiovascular illness
    c. The number of years since the first ever consumption of these nicotine-containing cigarettes
    d. Presence of nicotine addiction in his family and friends
19. Nicotine increases dopamine levels through inhibition of which of these enzymes?
    a. DOPA decarboxylase
    b. Aldehyde dehydrogenase
    c. Monoamine oxidase (MAO)
    d. Tyrosine hydroxylase
20. Which among the following is considered a gateway drug?
    a. Cocaine
    b. Heroin
    c. Tobacco
    d. Amphetamines
21. Nicotine patches are available in strengths of all of the following, *except*:
    a. 21 mg
    b. 14 mg
    c. 50 mg
    d. 7 mg
22. Which is the most common tobacco product used in smoking form in India?
    a. Clay pipe
    b. Cigarette
    c. Hookah
    d. Bidi
23. The following are symptoms of nicotine intoxication, *except*:
    a. Insomnia
    b. Excessive sedation
    c. Palpitation
    d. Psychomotor agitation

24. Which enzyme metabolizes nicotine into cotinine, a major nicotine metabolite?
    a. MAO
    b. Nicotine oxidase (NOX)
    c. Cytochrome P450 2A6 (CYP2A6)
    d. Acetylcholinesterase (AChE)

25. Tobacco withdrawal, according to DSM 5 (Diagnostic and Statistical Manual of Mental Disorders, 5th edition), includes all, *except*:
    a. Hypersomnia
    b. Increased appetite
    c. Depressed mood
    d. Restlessness

26. Which of the following statements is TRUE?
    a. Nicotine is well-absorbed in the stomach when the pH is acidic
    b. Nicotine is well-absorbed in the small intestine as the pH is alkaline
    c. Nicotine does not enter breast milk
    d. Nicotine is extensively metabolized in the lungs

27. In experimental research, the investigator is trying to assess the effectiveness of NRT in abstaining from tobacco use. Which of the following biomarkers can be used to find tobacco use by a person already on NRT?
    a. Cotinine
    b. Anabasine
    c. Trans-hydroxycotinine
    d. Trans-hydroxycotinine/cotinine ratio

28. Tobacco and nicotine cannot be used as ingredient in any food products in India based on _____
    a. Food Safety and Standards Regulations, 2011
    b. Drugs and Cosmetics Act, 1940
    c. Cigarettes and Other Tobacco Products Act (COTPA), 2003
    d. Cigarettes and Other Tobacco Products Amendment Rules, 2023

29. A person was found selling smokeless tobacco to a 10-year-old child. According to the Juvenile Justice (Care and Protection of Children) Act, 2015, what punishment is he liable to?
    a. Simple imprisonment of up to 3 years
    b. Rigorous imprisonment of up to 3 years
    c. Simple imprisonment of up to 7 years
    d. Rigorous imprisonment up to 7 years

30. The Food and Drug Administration (FDA)-approved NRTs include the following, *except*:
    a. Nicotine nasal spray
    b. Nicotine inhaler
    c. Nicotine vaccine
    d. Nicotine patch

31. The following NRT has been included in the National List of Essential Medicines, 2022?
    a. Nicotine patch
    b. Bupropion
    c. Varenicline
    d. Nicotine oral dosage forms

32. The WHO Model List of Essential Medicines contains all of the following, *except*:
    a. Nicotine spray
    b. Bupropion
    c. Nicotine inhaler
    d. Varenicline

33. This is a self-administered school-based survey of students aged 13–15 years to monitor tobacco use among youth, and developed as part of the Global Tobacco Surveillance System (GTSS).
    a. Global Student Tobacco Survey
    b. Global Youth Tobacco Survey (GYTS)
    c. Global Adolescent Tobacco Survey
    d. Global Middle School Tobacco Survey

34. The tobacco manufacturers employ various curing processes during tobacco production. The tobacco smoke from which curing process results in higher nicotine levels relative to others?
    a. Flue-curing
    b. Air-curing
    c. Fire-curing
    d. Sun-curing

35. The primary metabolite of nicotine, cotinine, is primarily formed through which enzymatic pathway in the liver?
    a. Glucuronidation
    b. Sulfation
    c. N-oxidation
    d. Methylation

36. FDA approved which neuromodulation modalities to aid smoking cessation?
    a. Deep transcranial magnetic stimulation
    b. Transcranial direct current stimulation
    c. Transcranial electrical nerve stimulation
    d. Vagus nerve stimulation

37. Which of the following is the major metabolite of nicotine, has low toxicity, and is often used as a biomarker for assessing nicotine exposure?
    a. Cotinine
    b. Nornicotine
    c. Nicotine-N'-oxide
    d. Nicotine-1'-N-oxide

38. A 30-year-old man with schizophrenia who has been symptom-free on haloperidol 20 mg for the past 5 years has recently quit smoking on the advice of his physician. He reports the emergence of rigidity and

tremors after stopping smoking. What is the most probable reason for the same?
   a. Decrease in the blood level of haloperidol
   b. Increase in the blood level of haloperidol
   c. Increase in nicotine levels leading to nicotine toxicity
   d. Decrease in nicotine levels leading to nicotine withdrawal
39. Nicotine exposure during pregnancy can adversely affect fetal development. Which of the following is a known risk associated with prenatal nicotine exposure?
   a. Decreased risk of sudden infant death syndrome (SIDS)
   b. Decreased risk of neural tube defects
   c. Lower risk of attention-deficit/hyperactivity disorder (ADHD)
   d. Increased risk of preterm birth
40. The EAGLES (Evaluating Adverse Events in a Global Smoking Cessation Study) found the following:
   a. There was a significant increase in neuropsychiatric adverse events in patients who took varenicline compared to nicotine patches
   b. There was a significant decrease in neuropsychiatric adverse events in patients who took varenicline compared to nicotine patches
   c. There was a significant increase in neuropsychiatric adverse events in patients who took varenicline compared to those who took a placebo
   d. There was no significant difference in the neuropsychiatric adverse events in patients who took varenicline compared to those who took a placebo
41. Which of the following is a known carcinogen in mint- or menthol-flavored e-cigarettes?
   a. Pulecone   b. Pulegone
   c. Pelegone   d. Pelecone
42. Cytotoxicity of e-liquid flavorings found toxicity to be greater in undifferentiated embryonic stem cells relative to:
   a. Human osteoblasts   b. Human pulmonary fibroblasts
   c. Human megaloblasts   d. Human erythroblasts
43. The sale of e-cigarettes is regulated to ensure quality and safety in:
   a. United Kingdom   b. Brazil
   c. Norway   d. Singapore
44. Varenicline is contraindicated in the following conditions, *except*:
   a. Renal impairment
   b. Hepatic impairment

c. Pregnancy
d. History of Stevens–Johnson syndrome with varenicline

45. The main constituents in the e-liquid include all, *except*:
    a. Propylene glycol
    b. Glycerol
    c. Ethyl alcohol
    d. Ethylene glycol

46. Which of the following is not true about Snus?
    a. Regulated as a food product under the Swedish Food Act
    b. Relatively low nicotine delivery and absorption than other smokeless tobacco
    c. Relatively lower levels of harmful substances
    d. Consumed by placing a pinch between the gum and upper lip

47. Which of the following is not true about heat-not-burn tobacco products?
    a. Disposable tobacco sticks
    b. Heated in an electronic device
    c. Produce aerosols containing nicotine and other chemicals by combustion
    d. Inhaled through the mouth

48. All of the following are true about heat-not-burn tobacco products, *except*:
    a. Processed tobacco is heated directly to produce vapor
    b. Processed tobacco is designed to be heated in a vaporizer
    c. Devices produce vapor from nontobacco sources, where the vapor is passed over processed tobacco to flavor the vapor
    d. Vapor is produced by heating nicotine liquid in a vaporizer

49. The first heat-not-burn tobacco product "Premier" was developed in 1988 by:
    a. British American Tobacco
    b. Japan Tobacco
    c. Imperial Tobacco Group
    d. RJ Reynolds

50. Brands of heat-not-burn tobacco products claimed all, *except*:
    a. Reduced secondhand smoke
    b. Reduced ash
    c. Reduced nicotine delivery
    d. Reduced smoke odor

51. All of the following are heat-not-burn tobacco products, *except*:
    a. Revo
    b. iQOS
    c. Vuse
    d. iFuse

52. Which of the following is not true regarding: In comparison with conventional cigarettes, heat-not-burn tobacco products have:
    a. Lower nicotine concentration in mainstream smoke
    b. Lower TSNAs (tobacco-specific nitrosamines)

c. Lower CO
d. Lower particulate matter

53. What is the amount of nicotine present in one conventional cigarette?
    a. 1–2 mg
    b. 10–14 mg
    c. 6–8 mg
    d. 20–24 mg

54. A 23-year-old female with a history of smoking cigarettes for the past 5 years came to you for help to quit. She reports significant craving and withdrawal symptoms whenever she attempts to quit the same. She also gives a history of seizure disorder, for which she has not taken any treatment currently. Which medication will you prefer in her case?
    a. No medication
    b. Nicotine-chewing gums
    c. Bupropion
    d. Varenicline

55. Which of the following is not true about heat-not-burn tobacco products?
    a. It needs to be inhaled within a few minutes, thus leading to nicotine peaks in the blood
    b. It leads to increased secondhand smoke release
    c. It causes intake of carbonyls, which are potential carcinogens
    d. It causes endothelial dysfunction similar to conventional cigarettes

56. Which of the following is found in much higher concentration in heat-not-burn tobacco products than conventional cigarettes?
    a. Acenaphthene
    b. Acrylamide
    c. Acrolein
    d. Acetaldehyde

57. E-cigarettes have been banned in India since:
    a. 2021
    b. 2022
    c. 2020
    d. 2019

58. Which of the following is NOT TRUE about the ban on e-cigarettes in India?
    a. The act was passed by the Ministry of Law and Justice
    b. All e-cigarettes, heat-not-burn tobacco products, and e-hookahs are banned
    c. It spares the electronic non-nicotine delivery system from the prohibition
    d. Punishment includes a 1-year jail term and ₹1 lakh fine

59. What is the prevalence of tobacco use in India according to the GATS 2 (2016–2017)?
    a. 24% in males and 12% in females
    b. 42% in males and 14% in females
    c. 34% in males and 18% in females
    d. 48% in males and 12% in females

60. Which of the following is not true about tobacco use in India?
    a. According to GYTS-4, 2019, more than half of students noticed anti-tobacco messages in mass media
    b. According to National Mental Health Survey (NMHS), 2016, the treatment gap for tobacco use is >90%
    c. According to GATS 2, current tobacco consumption is found in 24% of the population
    d. Bidi smoking is the most common form of tobacco-smoking

61. Which of the following is false about WHO-FCTC (World Health Organization–Framework Convention on Tobacco Control)?
    a. It was adopted at the 56th World Health Assembly
    b. It came into force on May 21, 2003
    c. It gives priority to the right to protect public health
    d. It includes cross-border effects in the tobacco epidemic

62. Which article of WHO-FCTC (World Health Organization–Framework Convention on Tobacco Control) promotes economically viable alternatives for tobacco worker growers?
    a. 15   b. 16
    c. 17   d. 25

63. Which of the following is true about WHO-FCTC (World Health Organization–Framework Convention on Tobacco Control)?
    a. It comprises 36 articles
    b. The US is a significant signatory to this treaty and has ratified it
    c. It only discusses preventing tobacco use and smoke exposure, with no support for reducing tobacco dependence
    d. It is the first global public health treaty

64. Which of the following is not true about the ban's effect on tobacco sales to minors?
    a. Tobacco use can decrease due to restricted access
    b. Tobacco use can decrease due to the "forbidden fruit effect"
    c. Tobacco use can continue due to access to noncommercial sources
    d. Tobacco use can continue if there are ways to circumvent the ban

65. Which of the following is not a part of the GTSS?
    a. GATS
    b. Global Student Tobacco Survey
    c. Global Health Professionals Student Survey
    d. Global School Personnel Survey

66. The GTSS was started by:
    a. WHO
    b. CDC (Centers for Disease Control and Prevention)

c. CPHA (Canadian Public Health Association)
d. All of the above

67. Percentage of adults who thought of quitting tobacco because of warning labels on packets according to GATS-2 is:
    a. Cigarettes > Bidi > Smokeless tobacco
    b. Bidi > Cigarettes > Smokeless tobacco
    c. Smokeless tobacco > Cigarettes > Bidi
    d. Bidi > Smokeless tobacco > Cigarettes

68. Which of the following legislations in India does not include tobacco-smoking?
    a. Motor Vehicles Act
    b. Drugs and Cosmetics Act
    c. Narcotic Drugs and Psychotropic Substances Act
    d. Cable Television Networks Amendment Act

69. COTPA Act includes all, *except*:
    a. Regulation of trade and commerce
    b. Regulation of production
    c. Regulation of supply and distribution
    d. Regulation of advertisement

70. Under Section 6 of the COTPA act, the sale of tobacco products is prohibited to individuals less than ___ years of age.
    a. 10   b. 16
    c. 18   d. 20

71. Which of the following is true for COTPA Act?
    a. It exempts a few states in India
    b. It does not include the power to add substance to a schedule
    c. The act also applies to tobacco products that are exported
    d. It specifies the size of letters and figures in the warning

72. The NTCP is run by the:
    a. Ministry of Health and Family Welfare (MOHFW)
    b. Ministry of Social Justice and Empowerment (MOSJE)
    c. Ministry of Finance
    d. Ministry of Home Affairs

73. Percentage of adults exposed to secondhand smoke according to GATS 2 is:
    a. Home > Workplace > Public place
    b. Workplace > Public place > Home
    c. Public place > Workplace > Home
    d. Public place > Home > Workplace

74. Which of the following statements is true about NRT in pregnancy?
    a. Good evidence is available to support the recommendation
    b. It should be considered when one is otherwise unable to quit
    c. A nicotine patch is preferred over intermittent NRT
    d. High-quality evidence shows that NRT alone is highly effective in abstinence during pregnancy

75. Breath CO level in nonsmokers is usually less than:
    a. 16 ppm
    b. 26 ppm
    c. 6 ppm
    d. 12 ppm

76. Kreteks include a mixture of tobacco and ___
    a. Areca nut
    b. Lime
    c. Clove
    d. Cardamom

77. Which of the following is not true about cotinine?
    a. The half-life is 8–30 hours
    b. It can be measured in urine only
    c. Screening can be done by immunological assay
    d. Confirmation needs to be done by chromatography

78. Which alkaloid can be tested specifically to detect recent tobacco use in people using electronic nicotine delivery systems (ENDS)?
    a. Anabasine
    b. Anatabine
    c. Nicotelline
    d. 4-(methylnitrosamino)-1-(3-pyridyl)-1-butanol (NNAL)

79. Which of the following is an ideal biomarker for secondhand exposure to nicotine?
    a. 4-(methylnitrosamino)-1-(3-pyridyl)-1-butanol
    b. Anabasine
    c. Anatabine
    d. Nicotelline

80. Which of the following is not being developed as a nicotine vaccine?
    a. NicVax
    b. TA-NIC
    c. NicPb
    d. Niccine

81. Off-label medications for tobacco dependence include all, *except*:
    a. Naltrexone
    b. Cytisine
    c. Sertraline
    d. Clonidine

82. NTCP has been merged with which program currently?
    a. National Tuberculosis Elimination Programme (NTEP)
    b. Drug De-addiction Programme (DDAP)

c. National Action Plan for Drug Demand Reduction (NAPDDR)
d. National Programme for Prevention and Control of Cancer, Diabetes, Cardiovascular Diseases and Stroke (NPCDCS)

83. Thirdhand smoke refers to _____
    a. Smoke inhaled by a smoker when he smokes a cigarette
    b. Smoke inhaled by a person near a smoker when the smoker smokes
    c. Residual smoke that remains on surfaces and dust after smoking tobacco
    d. Watching other people smoke on TV

84. The biomarker that helps to detect long-term exposure to tobacco is _____
    a. 4-(methylnitrosamino)-1-(3-pyridyl)-1-butanol (NNAL)
    b. Nicotine
    c. Breath CO level
    d. Cotinine

85. Which neurotransmitter system plays a significant role in nicotine withdrawal symptoms?
    a. Serotonergic system
    b. GABAergic system
    c. Noradrenergic system
    d. Cholinergic system

86. Oral contraceptives are contraindicated in women who smoke because of the following reasons, *except*:
    a. Greater risk of blood clots
    b. Greater risk of myocardial infarction
    c. Greater risk of bleeding
    d. Greater effectiveness of contraceptive pills

87. What is the approximate percentage of nicotine excreted unchanged in the urine after nicotine administration?
    a. <20%
    b. 20–40%
    c. 40–60%
    d. >60%

88. The chemical formula of nicotine is:
    a. $C_{10}H_{14}N_2$
    b. $C_{12}H_{10}N_2$
    c. $C_{14}H_{10}N_2$
    d. $C_{14}H_{12}N_2$

89. FTND stands for ____
    a. Fullerton Test for Nicotine Dependence
    b. Fish Test for Nicotine Dependence
    c. Finner Test for Nicotine Dependence
    d. Fagerström Test for Nicotine Dependence

90. According to the GYTS-4, the proportion of current tobacco users among students aged 13–15 years in 2019 was:
    a. 12.0%
    b. 8.5%
    c. 21.0%
    d. 14.6%

91. According to the GYTS-4, the proportion of students aged 13–15 years who thought other people's smoking was harmful to them in 2019 was:
    a. 30.5%
    b. 45.7%
    c. 50.3%
    d. 70.6%

92. Which of the following is true about nicotine vaccines?
    a. FDA has approved nicotine vaccine for smoking cessation
    b. Nicotine vaccine aims to elicit antibodies that block the pharmacological effects of nicotine
    c. Nicotine vaccine is a type of passive immunization
    d. Nicotine particles are large enough to induce the immune system

93. Elevated breath CO level in the absence of smoking can be due to all of the following, *except*:
    a. Use of smokeless tobacco
    b. Exposure to car exhaust
    c. Exposure to smog
    d. Exposure to clay ovens

94. Developing tolerance to nicotine's effects is a complex process involving both pharmacokinetic and pharmacodynamic mechanisms. Which of the following mechanisms contributes to pharmacodynamic tolerance?
    a. Desensitization of nicotinic receptors
    b. Downregulation of cytochrome P450 enzymes
    c. Increased nicotine metabolism
    d. Enhanced sensitivity of dopaminergic neurons

95. COTPA Act prohibits the sale of tobacco products within ____ yards of educational institutions.
    a. 10
    b. 20
    c. 50
    d. 100

96. The nicotinic acetylcholine receptor (nAChR) subunit cluster on chromosome 15 has been associated with the number of cigarettes smoked per day serum cotinine level, as the risk of lung cancer is;
    a. CHRNB1-CHRNB4-CHRNA1
    b. CHRNA5-CHRNA3-CHRNB4
    c. CHRNB1-CHRNA5-CHRNA1
    d. CHRNB1-CHRNB2-CHRNB3

97. The predominant enantiomer of nicotine found to occur naturally in tobacco is:
    a. S-enantiomer
    b. R-enantiomer
    c. A-enantiomer
    d. Z-enantiomer

98. GATS 2 is a household survey of persons with age more than or equal to _____ years.
    a. 12
    b. 14
    c. 15
    d. 18

99. FCTC stands for:
    a. Framework Convention on Tobacco Use
    b. Framework Convention on Tobacco Control
    c. Framework Convention of Tobacco Companies
    d. Framework Convention on Tobacco Challenges

100. The concept of "nicotine self-administration" is widely used in animal studies to model drug-seeking behavior and addiction. Which brain region is essential for the reinforcing effects of nicotine, as demonstrated in self-administration experiments?
    a. Ventral tegmental area (VTA)
    b. Hippocampus
    c. Thalamus
    d. Basal ganglia

ANSWER KEY

1. b	2. a	3. d	4. b	5. b	6. a	7. a	8. c
9. c	10. c	11. a	12. d	13. b	14. b	15. a	16. a
17. a	18. a	19. c	20. c	21. c	22. d	23. b	24. c
25. a	26. b	27. b	28. a	29. d	30. c	31. d	32. c
33. b	34. b	35. c	36. a	37. a	38. b	39. d	40. d
41. b	42. b	43. a	44. b	45. c	46. b	47. c	48. d
49. d	50. c	51. c	52. a	53. b	54. b	55. b	56. a
57. d	58. c	59. b	60. c	61. b	62. c	63. d	64. b
65. b	66. d	67. a	68. c	69. d	70. c	71. d	72. a
73. a	74. b	75. c	76. c	77. b	78. c	79. a	80. c
81. c	82. b	83. c	84. a	85. c	86. d	87. a	88. a
89. d	90. b	91. d	92. b	93. a	94. a	95. d	96. b
97. a	98. c	99. b	100. a				

FURTHER READING

1. Benowitz NL, Hukkanen J, Jacob III P. Nicotine chemistry, metabolism, kinetics and biomarkers. Nicotine Psychopharmacol. 2009;1:29-60.
2. El-Guebaly N, Carrà G, Galanter M, Baldacchino AM, (Editors). Textbook of addiction treatment: international perspectives. Springer Milan; 2015 Jan 26.
3. Miller S. The ASAM principles of addiction medicine. Lippincott Williams & Wilkins; 2018 Nov 26.
4. Prochaska JJ, Benowitz NL. The past, present, and future of nicotine addiction therapy. Annu Rev Med. 2016;67:467-86.
5. Tata Institute of Social Sciences (TISS), Mumbai and Ministry of Health and Family Welfare, Government of India. Global Adult Tobacco Survey GATS 2 India 2016-17.
6. Tata Institute of Social Sciences (TISS), Mumbai and Ministry of Health and Family Welfare, Government of India. Global Youth Tobacco Survey GYTS 4 India 2019
7. Yadav A, Singh PK, Yadav N, Kaushik R, Chandan K, Chandra A, et al. Smokeless tobacco control in India: policy review and lessons for high-burden countries. BMJ Glob Health. 2020;5(7):e002367.

CHAPTER 3

Cannabis

Rashmi Chakraborty, Sukriti Mukherjee, Aniruddha Basu

1. Which of the following cannabinoids is responsible for the psychoactive effects of cannabis?
   a. Cannabidiol
   b. Tetrahydrocannabinol (THC)
   c. Cannabinol (CBN)
   d. Dronabinol

2. Which of the following is not obtained from *Cannabis sativa*?
   a. Marijuana
   b. Hashish
   c. Bhang
   d. Heroin

3. The highest concentration of delta-9-THC is found in which part of the plant *C. sativa*?
   a. Leaves
   b. Roots
   c. Flowering tops
   d. Seeds

4. All of the following methods are commonly used for consuming cannabis, *except*:
   a. Smoking
   b. Vaporizing
   c. Oral ingestion
   d. Intravenous injections

5. THC exerts its effects on the brain by its action on the following receptor:
   a. Sigma receptor
   b. Cannabinoid type-1 (CB1) receptor
   c. Cannabinoid type-2 (CB2) receptor
   d. Serotonin receptor

6. Endogenous ligands of the cannabinoid signaling system in the brain is/are:
   a. Endorphin
   b. Enkephalin
   c. Anandamide
   d. All of the above

7. Which of the following is not seen in cannabis intoxication?
   a. Perceptual alteration
   b. Time distortion
   c. Pinpoint pupils
   d. Paranoid ideation

8. Which of the following statements is incorrect?
   a. There is evidence that cannabis use can precipitate schizophrenia in vulnerable individuals
   b. Cannabis use causes cognitive changes in the form of impaired short-term memory and attention

c. It does not cause withdrawal symptoms even after prolonged regular use
d. 2-arachidonoylglycerol (2AG) is an endogenous cannabinoid ligand

9. The following is not a feature of a motivational syndrome.
   a. It is commonly seen in recreational cannabis users
   b. It is characterized by a person's unwillingness to persist in any task requiring sustained attention and tenacity
   c. Tendency to become apathetic and anergic
   d. Whether the syndrome is solely related to cannabis use or reflects characterological traits/depressive features regardless of cannabis use is under debate

10. Which of the following is not a synthetic cannabinoid receptor agonist (SCRA)?
    a. Hash oil   b. Spice
    c. K2   d. JWH-018

11. As per the World Drug Report 2020, the risk of developing dependence on cannabis among those who have ever used the drug (even once) has been estimated (in studies conducted in the United States) at:
    a. 1%   b. 5%
    c. 9%   d. 20%

12. Which of the following is not correctly matched:
    a. Phytocannabinoid—2-AG
    b. Endocannabinoid—anandamide
    c. Synthetic cannabinoid (SCB)—dronabinol
    d. None of the above

13. A 19-year-old was brought to psychiatry outpatient department (OPD) the day after Holi by his family members with complaints of intense anxiety, talking irrelevantly, undue fearfulness, and complaining that people around him are mocking him while chatting among themselves. His vitals are afebrile, pulse 110 beats/min, and blood pressure (BP) 126/80 mm Hg. His urine drug screen is positive for THC. Noncontrast computed tomography (NCCT) head—nicotinamide adenine dinucleotide (NAD). Further history revealed that he had drunk around three to four glasses of "thandai" mixed with bhang the previous night. As per ICD-11 (International Classification of Diseases 11th Revision), his likely diagnosis will be:
    a. 6C41.3   b. 6C41.4
    c. 6C41.5   d. 6C41.6

52 Cannabis

14. In the scenario mentioned above, how will you manage the case?
    a. Offer him only a short course of benzodiazepine and follow-up after 7 days
    b. Start him on oral antipsychotic and follow up after a month
    c. Start him on selective serotonin reuptake inhibitor (SSRI) and follow up after a month
    d. Reassure him and send him home

15. A 35-year-old businessman with a history of long-standing daily use of cannabis was noted by his wife to behave oddly over the last week. He had stopped going to the office, complaining that an elaborate conspiracy was against him and that his colleagues were planning to kill him. He would put his hands to his ears and keep shouting and abusing alone in his room. On probing, he confided to his wife that through a transmitter fitted in his ear, he could capture the conversations of his colleagues in the office and communicate with them. Over the next week, he started refusing to eat and drink anything at home and would accuse his wife of ganging up with his persecutors to kill him. He was admitted to a mental institution and agreed having last used cannabis around 3 weeks back. As per ICD-11, his likely diagnosis will be:
    a. 6C41.3   b. 6C41.4
    c. 6C41.5   d. 6C41.6

16. How will you start to manage the case in this scenario mentioned above?
    a. Offer him only a short course of benzodiazepine and assess for symptoms for another week
    b. Start him on oral antipsychotic and assess for symptoms after a week
    c. Start him on SSRI and assess for symptoms after a week
    d. Start him on electroconvulsive therapy (ECT) and assess for symptoms after a week

17. A 25-year-old woman was brought to psychiatry OPD by her parents with complaints of muttering to herself, complaining that she could hear her neighbors discussing defaming her; she started neglecting her daily routine, became fearful of going out and remaining aloof and had withdrawn for the last 10 days. She had a similar episode around 2 years back, had improved with treatment, and had been asymptomatic without medications for the last 6 months. Her parents also informed her that for the last month, she had been partying with

friends where she had smoked weed twice or thrice. The preliminary working diagnosis would be:
   a. Cannabis-induced psychotic disorder
   b. Relapse of previous psychotic disorder
   c. Cannabis-induced mood disorder
   d. Cannabis withdrawal

18. After hitting his motorbike into an auto at a crossing while returning from a social gathering, the rider sustained bruises over his limbs and a small laceration on his forehead. The next morning, he went to a doctor who asked about his substance use. He denied consuming alcohol. His urine tested positive for THC. He admitted to having ganja with friends earlier that evening. He had smoked joints on a few earlier occasions but had never had any problems. In this case scenario, what would be his most appropriate diagnosis:
   a. 6C41.0
   b. 6C41.1
   c. 6C41.3
   d. He does not fulfill any diagnostic criteria for cannabis use

19. What would be the most appropriate management strategy for the above case?
   a. Admission to a drug rehabilitation center
   b. Structured motivational enhancement therapy (MET) sessions and cognitive behavioral therapy (CBT) for relapse prevention
   c. Brief intervention
   d. OPD management with pharmacotherapy

20. You plan to survey schools and colleges in your community for problematic cannabis use among adolescents and young adults. You decide to use a short screening tool that is not very extensive or time-consuming. Which of the following would NOT be a suitable screening tool?
   a. Marijuana Screening Inventory (MSI)
   b. Cannabis Abuse Screening Test (CAST)
   c. Cannabis Use Disorder Identification Test (CUDIT)
   d. Problematic Use of Marijuana (PUM)

21. A 24-year-old college student presents to the emergency after experimenting with drugs and has been diagnosed, as per ICD-11, with cannabis intoxication. Under ICD-11, which of the following criteria has not been included under cannabis intoxication:
   a. Perceptual alterations
   b. Impaired attention and judgment

54 Cannabis

  c. Conjunctival injection
  d. Suspiciousness or paranoid ideation

22. Under ICD-11, which of the following criteria has not been included under SCB intoxication?
    a. Delirium
    b. Acute Psychosis
    c. Nausea and vomiting
    d. Conjunctival injection

23. Which of the following statements is incorrect about cannabis withdrawal [292.0 of DSM-5 (Diagnostic and Statistical Manual of Mental Disorders, Fifth Edition)]?
    a. Most symptoms in criterion B have their onset within the first 24–72 hours of cessation, peak within the first week, and last approximately 1–2 weeks
    b. Any two or more symptoms from criterion B must be present that are not attributable to another medical condition and are not better explained by another mental disorder
    c. Physical symptoms may include loss of appetite, weight loss, abdominal pain, shakiness/tremors, sweating, fever, chills, or headache
    d. Rebound periods of increased appetite and hypersomnia may follow initial periods of loss of appetite and insomnia

24. A 26-year-old man reports to his family doctor that he has been using marijuana intermittently for relaxation and recreation since college. He has started using "herbal incense" and "Cloud 9" for the last year. Earlier, he was enjoying it, but he developed palpitations and dizziness and was noted to be argumentative and talking irrelevantly after smoking it. Recently, he needed to be taken to the emergency room because he had developed severe chest pain and breathing difficulty after one such episode. He had tachycardia, and BP was 166/96 mm Hg. His routine urine drug screen was negative. He was offered symptomatic management and, on improvement, sent back home. The most appropriate diagnosis would be:
    a. 6C42.1 Harmful pattern of use of synthetic cannabinoids
    b. 6C42.0 Single episode of harmful use of synthetic cannabinoids
    c. 6C42.3 Synthetic cannabinoid intoxication
    d. 6C42.4 Synthetic cannabinoid withdrawal

25. Which of the following is not covered under the Narcotic Drugs and Psychotropic Substances (NDPS) Act of 1985?
    a. Hashish
    b. Ganja
    c. Bhang
    d. Charas

26. Which of the following is not correct under the NDPS Act of 1985?
    a. The sale of preparations from leaves and seeds of female cannabis hemp plants is not a punishable offense
    b. Possession of small quantities of resin of hemp/cannabis plant for personal consumption of drugs is a punishable offense
    c. Section 10 of the NDPS Act allows states to permit and regulate the cultivation of any cannabis plant production, including charas
    d. The government may order the cultivation of cannabis plants for industrial purposes only for obtaining fiber or seed or for horticultural use

27. Sale, purchase, and possession of bhang is legal in all the following states, *except*:
    a. West Bengal
    b. Rajasthan
    c. Gujarat
    d. Assam

28. The following United Nations (UN) treaties regulate the medical and recreational uses of cannabis in most countries, *except*:
    a. 1961 Single Convention on Narcotic Drugs
    b. 1971 Convention on Psychotropic Substances
    c. 1988 Convention Against Illicit Traffic in Narcotic Drugs and Psychotropic Substances
    d. 1925 International Convention Relating to Dangerous Drugs

29. In 2021, based on World Health Organization scientific committee recommendations, the following changes in international law: Single Convention on Narcotic Drugs of 1961 was adopted:
    a. Removal of cannabis and cannabis resin from Schedule IV
    b. Addition of delta-9-THC to Schedule IV
    c. Addition of isomers THC to Schedule IV
    d. Downgraded cannabis and cannabis resin from Schedule IV to Schedule II

30. All of the following are approved medicinal use of cannabis by the US Food and Drug Administration, *except*:
    a. A synthetic THC (dronabinol) for treating chemotherapy-associated nausea and vomiting
    b. SCB, nabilone, for treating chemotherapy-associated nausea and vomiting and for stimulating appetite in patients with human immunodeficiency virus (HIV)
    c. Cannabidiol for treating two rare forms of seizures (Lennox-Gastaut and Dravet syndromes in young children and tuberous sclerosis from a benign brain tumor)
    d. Cannabidiol plus THC in a 1:1 ratio for treating multiple sclerosis (MS)-associated spasticity and neuropathic pain

31. Recreational use of SCBs, commonly available as "spice" and "K2", is an increasing public health problem globally. The following statements are INCORRECT:
    a. Acute intoxication with SCBs has been related to tachycardia, hypertension, nausea and vomiting, visual and auditory hallucinations, agitation and anxiety, and seizures
    b. JWH-018/JWH-073 is the psychoactive component of SCBs
    c. JWH-018 is a potent agonist at CB1 receptor and antagonist at CB2 receptors
    d. SCBs have a higher affinity for cannabinoid receptors than Δ9-THC

32. Laws regulating the manufacturing, commercial use, possession, import, and export of SCBs are covered under the following UN drug control conventions:
    a. Single Convention on Narcotic Drugs
    b. Convention on Psychotropic Substances
    c. Convention Against Illicit Traffic in Narcotic Drugs and Psychotropic Substances
    d. None of the above

33. In India, manufacturing, commercial use, possession, import, and export of SCBs are regulated under:
    a. Narcotic Drugs and Psychotropic Substances Act, 1985
    b. Narcotic Drugs and Psychotropic Substances (Amendment) Rules, 2015
    c. Notification GSR 899-E dated 23-12-2022—Narcotic Drugs and Psychotropic Substances Rules, 2022
    d. None of the above

34. A 21-year-old student was rushed to emergency after being found smoking "synthetic weed" in his hostel room. The patient was agitated and talking irrelevantly and had multiple episodes of vomiting. He had tachycardia and raised BP. Which of the following in this context is incorrect?
    a. Monitor for hypothermia
    b. Get a urine drug screen for THC
    c. Monitor for convulsions, myocardial infarction (MI), and arrhythmias
    d. Evaluate for acute kidney injury

35. SCBs have been classified into four distinct generations with different chemical structures. All of the following statements are correct, *except*:
    a. JWH-018 series belongs to the first generation and are potent CB1 agonists

b. THC has a higher affinity for CB1 and CB2 receptors than the first generation SCBs
c. Second- and third-generation SCBs have higher CB receptor affinity than the first generation
d. Current research indicates that due to the higher affinity for CB1 receptors and the lack of cannabidiol in SCRAs, they impose an increased risk of psychoses and schizophrenia

36. All of the following have been reported as adverse effects of SCRAs, except:
a. Neuropsychiatric—agitation, aggression, catatonia, paranoia, auditory and visual hallucinations, perceptual alterations, and psychosis episodes
b. Cardiovascular—tachycardia/bradycardia, hypertension, MI, arrhythmias, chest pain, and palpitations
c. Renal—acute kidney injury
d. Ocular—miosis

37. Amongst the following, which SCBs have the highest affinity for CB1 receptor?
a. JWH-018
b. HU-210 derivatives
c. AB-CHMINACA
d. THC

38. Detection and quantification of SCBs are challenging with the production of newer designer molecules in the market. Which of the following is the LEAST sensitive tool for detecting the latest-generation SCBs?
a. Immunoassays
b. Liquid chromatography–electrospray ionization–tandem mass spectrometry
c. High-resolution mass spectrometry
d. Gas chromatography–ion mobility spectrometry

39. Routine analytical approaches cannot monitor the new trends in the case of SCBs because when a substance is finally identified and incorporated into an analytical panel, its availability and use decrease. Out of the following, the most suitable technique to identify and quantify known and unknown SCBs and metabolites with high sensitivity and selectivity is:
a. Immunoassays
b. Liquid chromatography–electrospray ionization–tandem mass spectrometry
c. High-resolution mass spectrometry
d. Gas chromatography–ion mobility spectrometry

Cannabis

40. A 20-year-old girl had been smoking weed almost daily with friends. But recently, she was informed that the friend who used to supply it had run into trouble with the police. Soon, a friend offered her "legal weed" and called it "spice." She laced her e-cigarette with spice and smoked two to three of them. Suddenly, she started vomiting and felt dizzy and was noted to be shouting and cursing others, something she had never done earlier. When a friend tried to confront her, she got aggressive and started biting others. She was restrained and taken to the emergency department. There, she had an episode of seizures. On examination she was afebrile and her BP and pulse rate were moderately increased. Pupils were dilated. Her urine drug screen was negative; which of the following will be your most appropriate working diagnosis?
    a. Head trauma
    b. SCB intoxication
    c. Generalized tonic–clonic seizures (GTCS) with postictal confusion
    d. Schizophrenia

41. What would be the next suitable line of management?
    a. Loading dose of IV phenytoin
    b. Urgent NCCT head
    c. Symptomatic management with injectable benzodiazepines, IV fluids, antiemetics, and keeping her under observation
    d. Given a history of illicit drug use and aggressive behavior, inform the police

42. For patients of schizophrenia with a history of regular cannabis use, which of the following is NOT true?
    a. Patients who continue using cannabis are more likely to have adverse outcomes, including higher relapse rates, longer hospital admissions, and more severe positive symptoms than those who discontinue cannabis after the onset of psychosis
    b. Mendelian randomization studies suggest a causal effect of cannabis use on schizophrenia
    c. The magnitude of cognitive impairments associated with cannabis exposure does not tend to diminish after abstinence
    d. Reductions in cannabis use are a crucial intervention to improve outcomes in patients with psychosis

43. Which of the following statements is INCORRECT regarding cannabis use?
    a. THC does not cross the placenta in pregnant women
    b. Women frequently use cannabis during the antenatal period as self-medication for nausea and vomiting

c. Studies have demonstrated high odds of low birth weight in infants exposed to cannabis in utero
d. Women who used cannabis during pregnancy may have an increase in the odds of anemia compared with women who did not

44. As per the available results of ABCD (Adolescent Brain Cognitive Development) Study, a United States-based ongoing longitudinal research study, prenatal cannabis exposure (PCE) following maternal knowledge of pregnancy is associated with increased psychopathology during middle childhood. Significant associations have NOT been reported with which of the following compared to those without PCE?
    a. Rule-breaking and aggressive behavior and other conduct disorder symptoms
    b. Attention-deficit/hyperactivity disorder (ADHD) symptoms
    c. Somatic complaints
    d. Cognitive impairments like sluggish cognitive tempo and attention problems

45. A 54-year-old lady was given nabiximol for neuropathic pain. In her next review, she reported dizziness, nausea, and drowsiness. Which of the following is not an adverse effect of medicinal cannabis use?
    a. Depression   b. Anxiety
    c. Seizures   d. Constipation

46. Which of the following is NOT correct about medicinal cannabis use?
    a. Cannabidiol modulates the endocannabinoid system by enhancing anandamine levels, exacerbating psychotic symptoms
    b. Based on the GRADE (*Grading* of Recommendations, Assessment, Development, and Evaluation) approach, there was moderate-quality evidence to suggest that cannabinoids may be beneficial for treating chronic neuropathic or cancer pain
    c. There is some evidence for improvement in anxiety with cannabidiol
    d. Based on the GRADE approach, there is low-quality evidence for no effect of cannabidiol on psychosis

47. A 15-year-old boy began smoking "ganja" with friends at 15 years, and by the next 2 years, he was smoking five to six joints daily. The parents were concerned about his academic decline, rebellious behavior at home, and threatening to cut his wrist when disciplined by his father, leading them to seek psychiatric counseling. Early-onset use of cannabis in adolescent has been associated with:
    a. Increased odds of school/college dropout and job instability in young adulthood

b. Increased risk of self-harm behavior
  c. Higher probability of use of other illicit drugs
  d. All of the above

48. A 42-year-old man with chronic cannabis use presented to a physician for the third time in the last 5 months with complaints of severe nausea and multiple episodes of vomiting for 3–4 days, with pain and fullness in the epigastric region. He claimed inadequate relief with proton-pump inhibitor (PPI) and domperidone/metoclopramide. His wife reported that he was eating less, had been taking hot showers frequently, and claimed to be feeling better. What is his likely diagnosis?
  a. Gastroesophageal reflux syndrome
  b. Cyclical vomiting syndrome
  c. Cannabinoid hyperemesis syndrome
  d. Acute peptic ulcer

49. The most robust evidence for the management of the above case would be:
  a. Application of capsaicin cream to the abdomen
  b. Use of a 5HT3 antagonist
  c. Use of a dopamine antagonist
  d. Supportive management with fluid replacement, antiemetics, and cessation of cannabis

50. A 24-year-old man, using cannabis for the past 4–5 years on a recreational basis, developed a depressive episode with onset of symptoms within 2 days of last cannabis use. He argued in office and was suspended for 10 days. By the end of the third week, he had persistent, pervasive low mood, anhedonia, predominant pessimistic ideas, and disturbed biorhythms. He felt worthless for 4–5 days and contemplated ending his life. He was taken to a psychiatrist and started on SSRIs and other supportive management. His last cannabis use was before his suspension from office. After 3 weeks into treatment, his mother returned him to the doctor, complaining that he had become overactive and unusually argumentative. He was talking big most of the time, buying expensive items on loan, and if anybody opposed him, he would become angry and abuse them. He had resumed cannabis use in the last two days. His likely diagnosis is:
  a. Cannabis-induced mood disorder
  b. Medication-induced mood disorder
  c. Bipolar affective disorder
  d. Cyclothymic disorder

51. The most appropriate management strategy in the above case will be:
    a. Advice strict abstinence from cannabis and reassure the mother that the symptoms will improve with prolonged abstinence
    b. Stop SSRI and start a mood stabilizer/second-generation antipsychotic and inform the caregiver about the possibility of long-term pharmacological management and psychotherapy for cannabis use
    c. Emergency admission and ECT
    d. Start him on a cannabinoid receptor antagonist like rimonabant

52. A 24-year-old man, using cannabis for the past 4–5 years on a recreational basis, with no history of any psychiatric disorder, developed low mood, decreased energy, easy irritability, worries and tensions about office work, and decreased sleep and appetite, with onset of symptoms within 2 days of last cannabis use. He went to his family physician for some sleeping pills, who suggested a psychiatric consultation. He delayed his psychiatric consultation for 2 weeks. By then, his symptoms were persisting but waxing and waning. What would be the most suitable diagnosis?
    a. 6C41.70 Cannabis-induced mood disorder
    b. 6C41.71 Cannabis-induced anxiety disorder
    c. 6A70.0 Single episode depressive disorder, mild
    d. 6C41.4 Cannabis withdrawal

53. What would be the most appropriate management line per NICE (National Institute for Health and Care Excellence) guidelines for the above case?
    a. CBT and supportive psychotherapy for his symptoms, advising abstinence from psychoactive substances, and offering psychosocial interventions for cannabis use and follow-up
    b. SSRI, benzodiazepines, CBT for his symptoms, advice to abstain from psychoactive substances, and psychosocial interventions for cannabis use
    c. Strict abstinence from cannabis and follow up after 2 weeks
    d. Pharmacotherapy for cannabis dependence syndrome

54. Jatin, a 24-year-old college student, came to the university's health clinic seeking help for his cannabis use. He reported that he has been smoking cannabis daily for the past 2 years and has noticed that he struggles to concentrate on his studies and often feels anxious when not high. He has also experienced a decrease in motivation and has neglected some of his responsibilities. He is concerned about the impact of cannabis use on his academic performance and overall well-being.

62 Cannabis

What is the most appropriate initial step in managing Jatin's cannabis dependence?
a. Prescribe an anxiolytic medication for his anxiety symptoms
b. Refer him to a support group for individuals struggling with substance use disorders
c. Advise him to cut down his cannabis use gradually over the next few weeks
d. Recommend CBT to address his cannabis dependence and related issues

55. Saloni, a 30-year-old professional, has been using cannabis regularly for 5 years. She reports that she initially started using it recreationally but now needs to use larger amounts to achieve the same effects. Lately, on trying to cut down on her cannabis use, she gets irritability, insomnia, and difficulty concentrating. She is worried about the impact on her job performance and relationships.

What is the most appropriate pharmacological treatment option for Saloni's withdrawal symptoms?
a. Prescribe a long-acting benzodiazepine for a short duration
b. Start her on a gradually tapering regimen of oral cannabis
c. Recommend naltrexone to reduce cravings
d. Offer her a trial of bupropion

56. Alex is a 26-year-old graphic designer who has been using cannabis regularly for 4 years. He uses it to relax and unwind after work, but lately, he has noticed difficulty falling asleep and often wakes up feeling irritable. He has increased the amount of cannabis use to achieve the same relaxation. He came across a video about the potential harmful effects of cannabis on the brain. Now, he is seeking help to regain control over his cannabis use.

Which of the following approaches would be best suited here?
a. Buspirone along with CBT
b. Olanzapine along with CBT
c. Amitriptyline along with CBT
d. Chlordiazepoxide along with CBT

57. Lalita is a 29-year-old social worker using cannabis heavily for the past 7 years. She started using it recreationally with friends but gradually relied on it to cope with stress and anxiety. Lalita's dependence on cannabis has led to strained relationships with her family and difficulties in her professional life. She has sought treatment to overcome her cannabis dependence, and you started her on medication and CBT. She has maintained abstinence for the past

9 months and reports significant improvement in socio-occupational functioning.

How long will you continue the treatment?
a. Can plan for tapering off medication
b. Can plan for tapering off medication after 2 years
c. Can plan for tapering off medication after 5 years
d. Should continue the medication lifelong

58. Aisha, a 25-year-old woman, is 6 weeks' pregnant. She has been using cannabis regularly for the past 3 years to help manage her anxiety and insomnia. She is concerned about the potential impact of cannabis use on her pregnancy and the health of her developing baby.

    What is the most appropriate advice for Aisha regarding her cannabis use during pregnancy?
    a. It is safe for Aisha to continue using cannabis in moderation to manage her anxiety and insomnia during pregnancy
    b. Aisha should stop using cannabis immediately, as it can negatively affect the developing baby's brain and growth
    c. She can switch to using edibles instead of smoking cannabis, as it might be safer during pregnancy
    d. She should consult her healthcare provider about obtaining a prescription for medical cannabis to ensure safe use during pregnancy

59. Raj, aged 27 years old, was caught by the police with 100 g of cannabis during a routine check at a public event. He claims that he bought the cannabis for personal use and was not involved in any drug trafficking activities. Raj has no prior criminal record and works as a marketing executive.

    What legal consequences might Raj face for being caught in possession of 100 g of cannabis in India, given the circumstances?
    a. Raj might only face a fine, as the quantity is for personal use and he has no prior criminal record
    b. Community service and probation could be imposed, with the possibility of avoiding imprisonment
    c. Raj could face imprisonment for up to 6 months and a fine, per the NDPS Act
    d. Raj might be allowed to attend a mandatory drug education program without legal penalties

60. Dr Amit, a psychiatrist from a tertiary medical college, was approached by the local administration regarding a possible solution to the heavy

use of cannabis among adolescents in local villages. He schedules a training program for the community health officers (CHOs). Which of the following will be a better approach for the training program?
a. To encourage CHOs to intervene directly and counsel adolescents with cannabis use disorders
b. To educate CHOs about the potential benefits of cannabis use among adolescents
c. To equip CHOs with the skills to screen for cannabis use disorders and facilitate referrals for suspected cases
d. To encourage CHOs to investigate the matter and report to the police

61. Rita is a 29-year-old woman diagnosed with bipolar affective disorder. She has had multiple manic and depressive episodes in the past. For the last 15 days, she has been experiencing a manic episode with prominent psychotic features, including delusions of grandeur and auditory hallucinations. In addition, Rita has a comorbid history of cannabis dependence, and she admits to using cannabis regularly to cope with her mood swings. Her family members mentioned that she has been using cannabis throughout the day for the last 5 days and will become agitated if she is prohibited from using it. Her family is concerned about her erratic behavior and worsening symptoms.

    What is the most appropriate management approach for Rita?
    a. Initiate antipsychotic medication to address the psychotic symptoms and provide psychoeducation about the risks of cannabis use
    b. Focus on treating the manic episode with mood stabilizers and disregard the cannabis dependence for now
    c. Address the cannabis dependence first, as it might exacerbate the psychotic symptoms, and then initiate treatment for the manic episode
    d. Hospitalize Rita for immediate stabilization and cessation of cannabis use, followed by a combination of antipsychotics and mood stabilizers

62. Lina, a 28-year-old woman, has been using cannabis regularly for the past 8 years. She comes from a cultural background where cannabis use is considered a social activity common in religious ceremonies. Lately, her family members have noticed that her cannabis use impacts her physical health, work performance, and relationships. However, she is concerned that stopping cannabis may conflict with her cultural beliefs.

What is the most appropriate approach when managing Lina's cannabis dependence?
a. Recommend that Lina immediately quit cannabis to address her health and well-being, regardless of her cultural beliefs
b. Respectfully explore Lina's cultural beliefs and work with her to set achievable goals for reducing cannabis use
c. Provide Lina with a comprehensive plan for immediate abstinence from cannabis without discussing her cultural beliefs
d. Disregard Lina's cultural beliefs and focus solely on cognitive behavioral techniques for managing her dependence

63. Jamal is a 24-year-old man who used to take cannabis regularly. He quits using cannabis 1 month ago due to concerns about its impact on his mental health. However, Jamal has been experiencing an unusual phenomenon recently. Even though he is no longer using cannabis, he occasionally has vivid and intense episodes of feeling high on cannabis again. During these episodes, he experiences a distorted perception of time, heightened sensory perception, and a feeling of detachment from reality that he used to feel while using cannabis. These episodes happen without any apparent triggers and are distressing for him.

What term describes the phenomenon experienced by Jamal?
a. Dissociation
b. Deja vu
c. Flashback
d. Panic attack

64. Vivek is a 34-year-old man who has been using cannabis regularly for 5 years. He has always been a calm and introverted individual. One night, during a party, suddenly, his friends saw him taking a dagger in his hand and running toward his workplace, shouting the name of a certain colleague. He was intoxicated with cannabis at that moment. His friends somehow restrained him and brought him to the hospital. Three of his friends got injured during the process of restraining. He was sedated in the emergency. The next day, he could not recollect any events during that moment.

What term describes the phenomenon experienced by Vivek?
a. Flashback
b. Dissociation
c. Run amok
d. Depersonalization

65. Yatish is a 40-year-old man who has been struggling with both alcohol and cannabis dependence for several years. He experiences strong cravings for both substances and has made multiple attempts to quit, but he often relapses due to intense withdrawal symptoms and cravings. Yatish is motivated to overcome his substance dependence and is seeking effective treatment options.

Cannabis

Which pharmacological agent will you consider for managing alcohol and cannabis dependence in a patient like Yatish?
a. Baclofen
b. Fluoxetine
c. Disulfiram
d. Methadone

66. Pranjal is a 16-year-old boy struggling with cannabis use disorder for the last year. He smokes cannabis daily, negatively impacting his academic performance and relationships. Pranjal has tried to quit multiple times but finds it difficult to resist cravings, especially when he goes out for weekend parties with friends. He is determined to make a change and seeks help from a therapist.

    Which technique of therapy would best suit the case of Pranjal?
    a. CBT to explore the underlying causes of his cannabis use
    b. Dialectical behavior therapy (DBT) to enhance emotional regulation skills
    c. Craving management, refusal skills, and finding alternate pleasures to help him resist cravings and peer pressure
    d. MET to increase his motivation to quit cannabis

67. Manoj, a 23-year-old college student, has struggled with cannabis use disorder for 3 years. He smokes cannabis daily, which has led to poor academic performance, social isolation, and conflicts with family. Manoj acknowledges the negative impact of his cannabis use but finds it challenging to deal with stress due to academics. There were times when he had stopped taking cannabis for a few days, but eventually, the stress would get back to him. He mentioned that he does not know how to relieve stress.

    Which coping skill enhancement technique commonly used in CBT is relevant to help individuals like Manoj?
    a. Thought stopping
    b. Mindfulness meditation
    c. Exposure therapy
    d. ECT

68. Rahul, a 24-year-old business executive, has used cannabis regularly for the past few years. He started using cannabis to cope with transitioning from college to a full-time job. His parents have been through a difficult divorce, and he cannot accept the changes. His younger sister is struggling to adjust to the new dynamics, and there has been an increase in conflicts at home. His cannabis use has escalated, and he uses it all day on holidays to escape from the tension and avoid confrontations.

    Which family therapy approach is particularly relevant for addressing the case?
    a. Gestalt therapy
    b. Multidimensional family therapy (MDFT)

c. DBT
d. Rational emotive behavior therapy (REBT)

69. Nasir, aged 44 years old, presents to your clinic with a chronic cough attributed to regular cannabis use. He has been smoking cannabis daily for the past 6 years. Despite the persistent cough and concerns about his respiratory health, he strongly attaches to smoking weed and resists quitting. He states that cannabis helps him relax, alleviate stress, and enhance his creativity.

    Given Nasir's case, what is the most suitable management plan?
    a. Prescribing cough suppressant medication and recommending immediate cessation of cannabis use
    b. Providing informational pamphlets about the harmful effects of cannabis and encouraging abstinence
    c. Employing a combined approach of MET and CBT
    d. Scheduling regular checkups for monitoring the chronic cough without addressing cannabis use

70. Amiya, a 20-year-old college student, has been using cannabis heavily for the past 2 years. He used to be an active and motivated student, but recently, he has become lethargic and disinterested in studies and hobbies. He is unable to concentrate on his studies. He does not participate in college events like he used to do earlier. His grades have dropped, and he spends most of his time smoking cannabis and watching TV. He has started neglecting his roles and responsibilities at home and has lost touch with his friends. His friends are concerned about his behavior, and they brought him to the OPD for management.

    Given Amiya's case, what is the term used to describe the behavior seen in him?
    a. Withdrawal syndrome
    b. Amotivational syndrome
    c. Hyperactivity disorder
    d. Disinhibition syndrome

71. Manas is a 32-year-old man who has been successfully managed for schizophrenia with oral antipsychotic medication. He has been stable for the past few years, actively participating in therapy and adhering to his treatment plan. However, recently, he started smoking cannabis occasionally. He reports experiencing vivid hallucinations, paranoia, and increased schizophrenia symptoms during an intoxicated state, but otherwise, he is maintaining well when not intoxicated.

    Given his case, what is the most appropriate management plan for addressing the worsening of his schizophrenia symptoms after smoking cannabis?
    a. Encouraging him to quit taking his antipsychotic medication and replacing it with medical cannabis

b. Increasing the dosage of his oral antipsychotic medication to counteract the effects of cannabis
c. Providing psychoeducation about the risks of cannabis use in individuals with schizophrenia and offering support for quitting cannabis
d. Switching Manas to a different class of antipsychotic medication is more compatible with cannabis use

72. Daniel is a 38-year-old man struggling with cannabis dependence for several years. He has made multiple attempts to quit using cannabis, both on his own and with the help of treatment from addiction treatment facilities. However, he has been unable to abstain for over a few months.

    Given Daniel's case, what is the most appropriate management approach?
    a. Suggesting Daniel to stop trying to quit since his repeated attempts have been unsuccessful
    b. Recommending other psychoactive substances like alcohol to suppress his cravings
    c. Exploring Daniel's unique triggers, underlying psychological factors, and motivations and tailoring a comprehensive quit plan that combines pharmacological and non-pharmacological strategies
    d. Advising Daniel to rely exclusively on self-help materials and online resources to overcome his cannabis dependence

73. Malati, aged 25 years old, occasionally uses cannabis recreationally with her friends. Recently, she has noticed a significant increase in her appetite after using cannabis. After smoking or consuming cannabis, she often experiences intense hunger and cravings for unhealthy, calorie-dense foods. She eats larger portions and indulges in snacks she would not typically eat. What term describes this phenomenon of increased appetite and excessive eating after cannabis intake?
    a. Munchies
    b. Anorexia
    c. Bulimia
    d. Hyperorexia

74. Shakti is a 55-year-old man with a history of heavy alcohol consumption. He has been drinking heavily for the past 20 years, often consuming a large amount of alcohol daily. His family provided a history of Shakti consuming a heavy amount of cannabis over the past few days after facing a financial loss a week ago. Shakti came to the emergency with restlessness, irritability, and anxiety for 2 days after he was prohibited from taking substances. On examination, he was found to have severe confusion and disorientation. He was unable to recognize his family

members or his surroundings. His wife mentioned similar episodes in the past where Shakti would get better after 3–4 days but was unsure about the events around the episodes.

How will you manage the case?
a. Administer high doses of cannabis to alleviate his symptoms and gradually taper off its use
b. Monitor Shakti's condition and wait for the symptoms to subside independently, as they usually resolve after a few days
c. Begin immediate treatment with antipsychotic medication to manage his symptoms and stabilize his condition
d. Provide supportive care, ensure medical stabilization, and address the alcohol withdrawal and potential effects of cannabis use

75. Vikash is a 30-year-old man who exhibits heightened agitation, restlessness, and irritability once or twice every week, early in the morning. During these episodes, he often gets generalized muscle aches and pains, goosebumps, frequent yawning, runny nose, and sneezing. During these episodes, he paces around his living space, clenches his fists, and occasionally becomes confrontational with those around him. Vikash's family members are aware of his heavy and regular cannabis use. Interestingly, he consumes cannabis during these episodes to alleviate his distress, but the symptoms persist. Curiously, he would leave the area on his bike, returning approximately 30 minutes later, noticeably improved.

Given Vikash's case, what is the most suitable explanation for the recurrent episodes he experiences and his behavior during these episodes?
a. These are symptoms of cannabis withdrawal
b. These are symptoms of cannabis intoxication
c. These are symptoms of withdrawal from other substances like opioids
d. These are symptoms of hypoglycemic attacks

76. Rocky, a 25-year-old man, has been charged with a heinous crime committed while intoxicated with cannabis. He does not deny his presence at the scene but claims not to have any memory of the event due to his intoxication. He is a regular smoker of cannabis and was not forced to consume the substance. His defense attorney argues that he should be considered not guilty due to his claim of lack of memory and impaired cognitive functioning resulting from cannabis intoxication.

Which of the following sentences best describes his situation?
a. He can plead not guilty based on voluntary intoxication as he knowingly consumed cannabis

b. He cannot plead not guilty based on voluntary intoxication as it is not a valid defense under IPC (Indian Penal Code) Section 85
c. He can plead not guilty based on diminished capacity under IPC Section 85, as his cognitive functioning was impaired due to cannabis intoxication
d. He cannot plead not guilty based on automatism as it is not a recognized defense under IPC Section 86

77. Mohit is a 28-year-old man struggling with cannabis dependence for several years. His family members have performed several sacred rituals secretly to keep him abstinent. They have come to your clinic for his management and want to know about the nature of his addiction. As a doctor, what will you discuss regarding the nature of the illness to the family members?
    a. Cannabis addiction is a moral failing that results from weak willpower and poor decision-making
    b. The chemical properties of cannabis cause cannabis addiction and do not involve the brain
    c. Cannabis addiction is a complex brain disorder influenced by genetic, environmental, and neurological factors
    d. Cannabis addiction is a temporary phase that can be overcome through determination and self-discipline

78. Sadagopal, a 20-year-old college student, visited your clinic and mentioned that some classmates told him that cannabis is a cognitive enhancer and that taking a chillum of cannabis daily before studying would keep him focused on the study. He wants to know if it is true.

    What will you say to Sadagopal?
    a. Long-term cannabis use has no impact on memory functions
    b. Chronic cannabis use is associated with improved memory recall and cognitive abilities
    c. Chronic cannabis use can lead to memory impairments, particularly in attention, learning, and recall
    d. Long-term cannabis use enhances memory consolidation and leads to better retention of new information

79. Indubala, a 40-year-old woman, has MS for the past 15 years. She experiences severe muscle spasms, pain, and difficulty with mobility due to her condition. Despite trying various conventional treatments, she struggles with the debilitating symptoms. Her neurologist has discussed the potential use of medical cannabis.

    In this case, what is the primary rationale for considering medical cannabis as part of her treatment plan?
    a. Medical cannabis can cure MS and eliminate her symptoms

b. Medical cannabis can replace all other medications she takes for MS
c. Medical cannabis can potentially alleviate her severe muscle spasms, pain, and mobility difficulties
d. Medical cannabis will not impact her MS symptoms and should be avoided

80. Venkatesh, a 65-year-old man, has been living with advanced cancer for the past year. He undergoes chemotherapy and radiation treatments and experiences significant nausea, vomiting, and loss of appetite as side effects. His oncologist suggests considering medical cannabis.

    In this case, what is the primary purpose of using medical cannabis as part of his cancer treatment plan?
    a. Medical cannabis will replace chemotherapy and radiation treatments
    b. Medical cannabis can cure his cancer and eliminate the need for further treatments
    c. Medical cannabis will specifically target cancer cells and halt their growth
    d. Medical cannabis can help alleviate treatment-related symptoms such as nausea, vomiting, and loss of appetite

The consumption of cannabis directly targets the endocannabinoid system of the brain. A new psychiatry resident starts reading about the endocannabinoid system and finds some interesting facts about it. Please answer the following three questions based on the unique features of the endocannabinoid system:

81. There are two types of receptors: CB1 and CB2. CB1 is mostly present in the following areas, *except*:
    a. Basal ganglia   b. Hippocampus
    c. Amygdala   d. Spinal cord

82. CB2 receptors are mostly present in which of the following?
    a. Basal ganglia   b. Immune cells
    c. Amygdala   d. Hippocampus

83. Transsynaptic transmission in the endocannabinoid system is:
    a. Anterograde   b. Retrograde
    c. Forward   d. Fast forward

Scenario: A 30-year-old male presents to the outpatient department of an addiction treatment facility with a history of over 10 years of cannabis use. Based on this case scenario, answer the following two questions:

Cannabis

84. Magnetic resonance imaging (MRI) studies reveal that grey matter volume is reduced in all the brain areas, *except*:
    a. Cerebellum
    b. Striatum
    c. Amygdala
    d. Hippocampus

85. His chronic drug-seeking is mostly attributed to impaired decision-making, related to which of the following?
    a. Decreased cholinergic transmission
    b. Decreased glutamatergic transmission
    c. Decreased serotonergic transmission
    d. Decreased dopaminergic transmission

Scenario: A new resident in the addiction treatment clinic evaluates a youth with cannabis dependence and finds several family members are using cannabis and other substances. For this case scenario, please answer the following three questions:

86. About the genetic liability of cannabis use versus cannabis dependence:
    a. Use = Dependence
    b. Use > Dependence
    c. Dependence > Use
    d. Neither dependence nor use has any genetic liability

87. One of his brothers, an early teenager, undergoes neuroimaging and has a reduced orbitofrontal cortex (OFC) volume. This is predictive of:
    a. Cannabis-related hypersensitivity
    b. Protection against cannabis use
    c. Initiation of cannabis use in later adolescence
    d. Cannabis-related cognitive decline

88. The patient underwent functional imaging and was found to have a chronic reduction in the CB1 receptor. On getting this feedback, he stopped cannabis use. This usually leads to the following changes in the CB1 receptor:
    a. Permanent reduction in the number of CB1 receptors
    b. Immediate normalization
    c. Normalization within a few weeks
    d. No change in the CB1 receptor system

Scenario: A neuroscience laboratory researching cannabis addiction plans to study the shift from goal-directed to habitual behaviors. In this regard, please answer the following two questions:

89. During habitual/compulsive drug-seeking behavior, which structures are involved?
    a. Basolateral amygdala
    b. Dorsal striatum
    c. Nucleus accumbens shell
    d. Nucleus accumbens core

90. To study the shift from goal-directed to habitual behaviors, which of the following paradigms will you choose?
    a. Devaluation paradigm
    b. Place preference paradigm
    c. Forced swim test paradigm
    d. Drug discrimination models

91. Studies that used chemogenetic tools like Designer Receptors that were exclusively activated by Designer Drugs (DREADD) or deactivated via knockout mice have found which neurocircuit enhances habitual behaviors.
    a. OFC and ventral striatum
    b. OFC and dorsomedial striatum
    c. OFC and thalamocortical junction
    d. Dorsolateral prefrontal cortex (DLPFC) and nucleus accumbens

92. You plan to study drug cue-induced over-potentiation in a molecular science laboratory. Due to their involvement, you may plan to study some of the following, *except*:
    a. Glutamate transporter 1 (GLT-1), which removes glutamate from the synaptic cleft
    b. Metabotropic glutamate receptor 5 (mGluR5), a receptor found in interneurons, which expresses neuronal nitric oxide synthase
    c. Matrix metalloproteinase 9 (MMP9) that causes local degradation of extracellular matrix
    d. Kappa receptor activation

93. If you plan to replicate a model emphasizing "the dark side of addiction", which of the following is true about the neuromodulator dynorphin?
    a. Dynorphin is a µ-opioid whose expression is modulated by activating dopamine or opioid receptors
    b. Kappa opioids induce feelings of euphoria
    c. Compulsive drug taking increases dynorphin levels in the nucleus accumbens and amygdala
    d. Injecting a kappa antagonist into the dynorphin-expressing areas of the nucleus accumbens increases excessive drinking in alcohol-dependent rats

94. To understand better the neuroscience of addiction, you plan to work on a computational model of dopamine release in response to rewards and expectations. You try to find the neural signatures associated with fictive errors. Using functional MRI (fMRI), you found that the following structures were involved, *except*:
    a. Ventral caudate
    b. Ventral putamen
    c. Insula
    d. Posterior parietal cortex

Cannabis

95. You plan to study the endocannabinoid system. Which of the following would you target?
    a. N-arachidonoylethanolamine (AEA) & 2-arachidonoylglycerol (2-AG) binding with receptors in the postsynaptic neuron
    b. AEA and 2-AG binding with receptors in the presynaptic neuron
    c. A drug mimicking cannabidiol
    d. A drug with structural and functional similarity with cannabidiol

96. You plan to study the effects of dopamine in the brain on addiction. Which of the following is TRUE concerning the dopamine receptors in the brain?
    a. D1 receptors have an approximately 10- to 100-fold greater affinity for dopamine than D2 receptors
    b. D2 receptors have an approximately 10- to 100-fold greater affinity for dopamine than D1 receptors
    c. Addicted individuals have a reduction in D2 receptors and increased dopamine activity in the OFC, anterior cingulated gyrus, and DLPFC areas
    d. D1 receptors are activated at higher dopamine concentrations compared to D2 receptors

97. You plan to study the brain's default mode network and its relationship with addiction. In this regard, you must study the resting state functional connectivity (rsFC). The following analytical approaches are used in the rsFC, *except*:
    a. Seed-based analysis
    b. Independent component analysis
    c. Diffusion tensor imaging
    d. Density mapping

98. A gentleman who has severe cannabis and tobacco (smoking) dependence had a road traffic accident and suffered from a traumatic brain injury. After that, he reported hardly appreciating the cannabis and tobacco smoke. Which areas of the brain may be involved?
    a. Amygdala
    b. Area postrema
    c. Ventral tegmental area (VTA)
    d. Insula

99. In your neuroscience research, you learned that habenula is one of the important structures mediating addiction. Which is one of the important neuromodulators in habenula?
    a. Dynorphin
    b. Acetylcholine
    c. Glutamate
    d. Corticotrophin-releasing peptide

100. As a neuroscientist working with neuroimaging, you plan to do neuroimaging related to the four interconnected neurocircuits of i-RISA. Under such circumstances, you will focus upon the following, *except*:
   a. Mood
   b. Reward
   c. Executive control
   d. Motivation drive

ANSWER KEY

1. b	2. d	3. c	4. d	5. b	6. c	7. c	8. c
9. a	10. a	11. c	12. a	13. a	14. a	15. d	16. a
17. b	18. a	19. c	20. a	21. d	22. c	23. b	24. a
25. c	26. c	27. d	28. d	29. a	30. d	31. c	32. d
33. d	34. b	35. b	36. d	37. c	38. a	39. c	40. b
41. c	42. c	43. a	44. c	45. d	46. a	47. d	48. c
49. d	50. c	51. b	52. a	53. a	54. d	55. a	56. a
57. a	58. b	59. c	60. c	61. d	62. b	63. c	64. c
65. a	66. c	67. b	68. b	69. c	70. b	71. c	72. c
73. a	74. d	75. c	76. b	77. c	78. c	79. c	80. d
81. d	82. b	83. b	84. a	85. b	86. c	87. c	88. c
89. b	90. a	91. b	92. d	93. c	94. c	95. b	96. c
97. c	98. d	99. a	100. a				

FURTHER READING

1. Alves VL, Gonçalves JL, Aguiar J, Teixeira HM, Câmara JS. The synthetic cannabinoids phenomenon: from structure to toxicological properties. A review. Crit Rev Toxicol. 2020;50(5):359-82.
2. Baranger DAA, Paul SE, Colbert SMC, Karcher NR, Johnson EC, Hatoum AS, et al. Association of Mental Health Burden With Prenatal Cannabis Exposure From Childhood to Early Adolescence: Longitudinal Findings From the Adolescent Brain Cognitive Development (ABCD) Study. JAMA Pediatr. 2022;176(12): 1261-5.
3. Basu D, Dalal PK. Overview of IPS Guidelines 2014. In: Basu D, Dalal PK (Eds). Clinical Practice Guidelines for the Assessment and Management of Substance Use Disorders. New Delhi: Indian Psychiatric Society; 2014; pp. 1-12.
4. Black N, Stockings E, Campbell G, Tran LT, Zagic D, Hall WD, et al. Cannabinoids for the treatment of mental disorders and symptoms of mental disorders: a systematic review and meta-analysis. Lancet Psychiatry. 2019;6(12):995-1010. Erratum in: Lancet Psychiatry. 2020;7(1):e3.
5. Eytan A. From running amok to mass shootings: a psychopathological perspective. Rev Med Suisse. 2019;15(663):1671-4.
6. Ferland JM, Hurd YL. Deconstructing the neurobiology of cannabis use disorder. Nature Neuroscience. 2020;23(5):600-10.

7. Lac A, Luk JW. Testing the Amotivational Syndrome: Marijuana Use Longitudinally Predicts Lower Self-Efficacy Even After Controlling for Demographics, Personality, and Alcohol and Cigarette Use. Prev Sci. 2018;19(2):117-26.
8. Murthy P, Dhawan A, Basu, D, Gupta M, Chandra M, Chand PK, et al. Standard Treatment Guidelines for managing Substance Use Disorders and Behavioural Addictions. New Delhi: Tobacco Control and Drug De-Addiction Programme, Ministry of Health and Family Welfare, Government of India; 2020.
9. National Institute on Drug Abuse. (2023). Cannabis (Marijuana) Research Report References. website. [online] Available from https://nida.nih.gov/publications/research-reports/marijuana/references [Last accessed December, 2023].
10. Sadock BJ, Sadock VA, Ruiz P. Kaplan and Sadock's Comprehensive Textbook of Psychiatry, 10th edition. Philadelphia: Wolters Kluwer; 2017.
11. Tait RJ, Caldicott D, Mountain D, Hill SL, Lenton S. A systematic review of adverse events arising from the use of synthetic cannabinoids and their associated treatment. Clin Toxicol (Phila). 2016;54(1):1-13.
12. Verweij KJ, Zietsch BP, Lynskey MT, Medland SE, Neale MC, Martin NG, et al. Genetic and environmental influences on cannabis use initiation and problematic use: a meta-analysis of twin studies. Addiction. 2010;105(3):417-30.
13. Whiting PF, Wolff RF, Deshpande S, Di Nisio M, Duffy S, Hernandez AV, et al. Cannabinoids for Medical Use: A Systematic Review and Meta-analysis. JAMA. 2015;313(24):2456-73. Erratum in: JAMA. 2015;314(8):837. Erratum in: JAMA. 2015;314(21):2308. Erratum in: JAMA. 2016;315(14):1522.
14. World Health Organization. International Classification of Diseases, Eleventh Revision (ICD-11). [online] Available from https://icd.who.int/en [Last accessed November, 2023].

CHAPTER 4

Opioids

Amit Singh, Arpit Parmar, Rahul Mathur

1. A state of acute opioid dependence can be noticed in humans after the administration of opioids at least:
   a. One time
   b. Seven times
   c. 14 times
   d. 21 times
2. High intensity and sensitivity to negative emotional states associated with opioid withdrawal is:
   a. Hyperpathia
   b. Hyperkatifeia
   c. Dysphoria
   d. Dysesthesia
3. Which of the following statements about buprenorphine is wrong?
   a. It is a synthetic opioid
   b. It is derived from thebaine
   c. It is a partial opioid agonist
   d. It has an elimination half-life of 2–6 hours.
4. Which of the following is not enlisted in the Government of India notification, 2015, as an "essential narcotic drug"?
   a. Codeine
   b. Methadone
   c. Buprenorphine
   d. Fentanyl
5. The "commercial quantity" of tramadol, as per the Narcotic Drugs and Psychotropic Substances (NDPS) Act 1985, is:
   a. 5 g
   b. 50 g
   c. 150 g
   d. 250 g
6. The Government of India does NOT permit licit opium poppy cultivation in this state.
   a. Madhya Pradesh
   b. Uttar Pradesh
   c. Rajasthan
   d. Haryana
7. Which of the following nations is not a part of the "Golden Triangle" region of the opium economy?
   a. Myanmar
   b. Cambodia
   c. Laos
   d. Thailand
8. Which of the following nations is not a part of the "Golden Crescent" region of the opium economy?
   a. Iran
   b. Afghanistan
   c. Pakistan
   d. Turkmenistan

Opioids

9. Methadone maintenance treatment for the treatment of opioid use disorder was introduced by:
    a. Dole and Nyswander
    b. Finnegan
    c. Edward Khantzian
    d. Kidorf and Hollander

10. Buprenorphine is preferable to methadone for opioid maintenance treatment due to all of the following, *except*:
    a. Due to less adverse effects
    b. Due to less drug–drug interactions
    c. In patients with a high risk for treatment dropout
    d. Facilitate safer take-home dosing

11. In buprenorphine maintenance treatment, the target dose of buprenorphine should be:
    a. Sufficient to produce the opioid-blocking effect
    b. Sufficient to stop withdrawals
    c. Sufficient to control craving
    d. 4 mg

12. Peak heroin withdrawal occurs at ... hours after last dose.
    a. 8–12 hours
    b. 12–20 hours
    c. 20–36 hours
    d. 48–72 hours

13. Which of the following indicates suitability for antagonist treatment in opioid use disorder?
    a. Injecting drug use
    b. Opioid use for 3 months
    c. Comorbid psychiatric illness
    d. Poor motivation

14. Commercial quantity of morphine/heroin as per NDPS Act is
    a. 250 g
    b. 500 g
    c. 1,000 g
    d. 2,500 g

15. Laudanum contains:
    a. Opium
    b. Cocaine
    c. Cannabis
    d. Nicotine

16. Confessions of an English Opium-eater book was written by:
    a. Thomas De Quincey
    b. Friedrich Sertürner
    c. Elizabeth Barrett Browning
    d. Vincent P. Dole

17. The opioid overdose triad has all, *except*:
    a. Pinpoint pupils
    b. Unconsciousness
    c. Depressed respiration
    d. Shock

18. The highest prevalence of blood-borne viruses in people who inject drugs is of:
    a. Human immunodeficiency virus (HIV)
    b. Hepatitis B virus (HBV)

c. Hepatitis C virus (HCV)
d. Herpes

19. United States Food and Drug Administration (US FDA)-approved medication for the management of opioid withdrawal is all, *except*:
    a. Methadone
    b. Lofexidine
    c. Clonidine
    d. Buprenorphine

20. Which of the following is not a feature of opioid intoxication?
    a. Yawning
    b. Drooping eyelids
    c. Scratching
    d. Head nodding

21. Which of the following is false about ultrarapid opioid detoxification?
    a. Guidelines recommend against its use in the treatment of opioid withdrawal
    b. Anesthesia is used
    c. Diuretic is used
    d. Small doses of naloxone are used

22. As per the National Survey on Extent and Pattern of Substance Use in India, 2019, the prevalence of opioid use in India is:
    a. 2.8%
    b. 2.1%
    c. 0.26%
    d. 0.25%

23. The opioid used most commonly for injecting by people who inject drugs is:
    a. Buprenorphine
    b. Pentazocine
    c. Tramadol
    d. Fentanyl analogs

24. Which of the following is incorrect about neonatal abstinence syndrome (NAS)?
    a. Characterized by central nervous system (CNS) and gastrointestinal (GI) and respiratory disturbances
    b. The modified Finnegan scale is used for monitoring
    c. Phenobarbitone is used for treatment
    d. Morphine should not be used for treatment

25. Identify the incorrect statement regarding the use of buprenorphine for maintenance treatment during pregnancy, as compared to methadone.
    a. Mothers treated with buprenorphine had shorter hospital stays
    b. Mothers treated with buprenorphine are less likely to drop out of treatment
    c. Infants born to mothers on buprenorphine have shorter treatment durations for NAS
    d. A lower cumulative dose of morphine is required to manage NAS

Opioids

26. According to the National Policy on Narcotic Drugs and Psychotropic Substances, which of the following is incorrect?
    a. Needle and syringe distribution should not be allowed in prisons
    b. Opioid substitution therapy should not be allowed in prisons
    c. No drug injector should be allowed opioid substitution therapy beyond 3 years
    d. Encouraging people with opioid addiction to smoke instead of injecting is not allowed

27. According to the NDPS Act of 1985, a preparation of coagulated opium poppy juice containing 0.1% morphine is termed:
    a. Opium
    b. Opium derivative
    c. Prepared opium
    d. Poppy straw

28. Tolerance develops for which feature of opioids?
    a. Miosis
    b. Constipation
    c. Convulsions
    d. Cough suppression

29. Incorrect statement about the Clinical Opiate Withdrawal Scale is:
    a. It has 10 items
    b. Tremor is one of the items
    c. A score of >36 indicates severe withdrawal
    d. Consciousness is not an item on the scale

30. The concentration of morphine in poppy straw is about:
    a. 0.01%
    b. 0.1%
    c. 1%
    d. 10%

31. The concentration of morphine in air-dried opium gum is:
    a. 0.01%
    b. 0.1%
    c. 1%
    d. 10%

32. Which of the following about poppy seeds is incorrect?
    a. Poppy seeds contain no morphine
    b. They contain no methadone
    c. Seeds are kidney-shaped
    d. They are popularly known as khuskhus in India

33. Skin popping refers to subcutaneous or intradermal injection of:
    a. Morphine
    b. Cocaine
    c. Hashish oil
    d. Mephedrone

34. The lowest potential for seizure is in:
    a. Meperidine
    b. Fentanyl
    c. Pentazocine
    d. Buprenorphine

35. Possible etiology for stroke in opioid users includes all, *except*:
    a. Vasculitis
    b. Hypotension
    c. Secondary to peripheral vasoconstriction
    d. Positional vascular compression

36. Which of the following opioid peptides has the highest affinity for κ (kappa) receptor?
    a. Dynorphins
    b. Endorphins
    c. Met-enkephalins
    d. Leu-enkephalins

37. Opioids stimulate the release of all of the following, *except*:
    a. Antidiuretic hormone (ADH)
    b. Prolactin
    c. Somatotropin
    d. Luteinizing hormone (LH)

38. Which of the following is incorrect about diphenoxylate?
    a. It is used to treat diarrhea
    b. A combination with atropine is often used
    c. Dependence may develop for it
    d. It does not cross the blood–brain barrier

39. Peripheral enteric μ-receptor antagonism and minimal CNS penetration are not the features of:
    a. Loperamide
    b. Methylnaltrexone
    c. Alvimopan
    d. Naloxegol

40. Tramadol intoxication is not associated with:
    a. Seizures
    b. Serotonin syndrome
    c. Respiratory depression
    d. Increased LH release

41. Morphine depresses respiration by:
    a. Direct depressant effect on intrinsic rhythm generators located in the ventrolateral medulla
    b. Depression of the ventilatory response to increased CO_2
    c. Effect on carotid and aortic body chemosensors
    d. All of the above

42. Psychotomimetic effect is least noticeable with:
    a. Morphine
    b. Nalorphine
    c. Butorphanol
    d. Pentazocine

43. What is the ratio of buprenorphine and naloxone in the commercially available buprenorphine–naloxone combination?
    a. 1:1
    b. 2:1
    c. 3:1
    d. 4:1

Opioids

44. Which of the following best reflects the relative efficacy of opioids in pain states?
    a. Tissue injury > acute stimuli = nerve injury = 0
    b. Tissue injury = acute stimuli ≥ nerve injury > 0
    c. Nerve injury > tissue injury = acute stimuli = 0
    d. Nerve injury ≥ tissue injury > acute stimuli = 0

45. In India, HIV prevalence (%) is highest in which population group?
    a. People who inject drugs
    b. Commercial sex workers
    c. Men who have sex with men (MSM)
    d. Transgender

46. Which of the following Harm reduction services is unavailable in India?
    a. Needle and syringe programs
    b. Condom distribution
    c. Drug consumption room
    d. Outreach and education

47. Which drug is used most commonly for opioid substitution therapy worldwide?
    a. Methadone
    b. Buprenorphine
    c. Diamorphine
    d. Slow-release oral morphine (SROM)

48. Which of the following medications is not indicated for opioid dependence in pregnancy?
    a. Methadone
    b. Buprenorphine
    c. Naltrexone
    d. None of the above

49. Which of the following is not a characteristic of low-threshold buprenorphine treatment?
    a. Same-day treatment entry prescription at first visit
    b. Reduced visit frequency based on clinical stability
    c. Reduction in illicit opioid use as an acceptable goal
    d. Programmatic rules prioritized

50. True about injectable naltrexone depot in opioid dependence is
    a. Reduces heroin use
    b. Reduce relapse rates
    c. More time spent in treatment
    d. No risk of opioid overdose

51. Speedball is a mixture of:
    a. Cocaine and heroin
    b. Cocaine and caffeine
    c. Cocaine and methylphenidate
    d. Cocaine and amphetamine

52. The states of opiate intoxication after administering 1 mg heroin follows this sequence:
    a. Nod → rush → high → being straight
    b. Being straight → rush → high → nod
    c. Rush → nod → being straight → high
    d. Rush → high → nod → being straight

53. The dopaminergic neurotransmitter system is implicated in opioid use disorders in the following way:
    a. It is the central neurotransmitter that mediates reward
    b. Dopamine D2/3 receptor availability is enhanced
    c. Presynaptic dopamine release is enhanced in heroin-dependent subjects
    d. All of the above

54. The heritability estimate of opioid addiction is:
    a. 10%
    b. 30%
    c. 50%
    d. 75%

55. A single spray of the FDA-approved NARCAN® nasal spray delivered by intranasal administration into one nostril delivers ...... of naloxone hydrochloride.
    a. 0.4 mg
    b. 1 mg
    c. 4 mg
    d. 8 mg

56. Analysis of this biological material can provide information about morphine use a month back.
    a. Urine
    b. Saliva
    c. Hair
    d. Blood

57. Pseudoaddiction is a phenomenon common in:
    a. Sickle cell disease
    b. Depression
    c. Mania
    d. Hepatosteatosis

58. Chest wall rigidity is most common with:
    a. Sufentanil
    b. Pethidine
    c. Morphine
    d. Methadone

59. The risk of torsades de pointes is highest with:
    a. Pentazocine
    b. Tramadol
    c. LAAM (levo-alpha-acetylmethadol)
    d. Codeine

60. The agonist effect produced by buprenorphine is around ...... of the maximum effect produced by opioid agonist.
    a. 10%
    b. 50%
    c. 70%
    d. 90%

Opioids

61. Which of the following is not synthesized from thebaine?
    a. Buprenorphine
    b. Naltrexone
    c. Oxymorphone
    d. Tramadol

62. Heroin is controlled under which schedule of the Single Convention on Narcotic Drugs?
    a. I
    b. II
    c. IV
    d. I and IV

63. Which of the following statements is incorrect?
    a. Heroin is more potent than morphine
    b. Heroin acts faster than morphine
    c. Heroin acts for a longer duration than morphine
    d. None of the above

64. The duration of action of buprenorphine is the longest for:
    a. Oral route
    b. Sublingual route
    c. Intramuscular route
    d. Intravenous route

65. Buprenorphine is contraindicated in patients with:
    a. Known hypersensitivity to buprenorphine
    b. Hepatitis
    c. Renal failure
    d. All of the above

66. A 60-year-old man with a long history of GI adhesions and chronic pancreatitis presents to the emergency room with stomach pain. The patient was given medication for pain. Minutes later, he has a tonic-clonic seizure. Which of the following opioid analgesics is most likely to have caused this patient's presentation?
    a. Naltrexone
    b. Pethidine
    c. Codeine
    d. Oxycodone

67. Which of the following opioids is associated with the highest level of immunosuppression?
    a. Morphine
    b. Tramadol
    c. Hydromorphone
    d. Buprenorphine

68. The formulations to prevent the diversion of opioids include all, *except*:
    a. Combining the opioid agonist with an antagonist
    b. Delivering the opioid in a readily extractable form
    c. Combining the opioid with a substance that triggers an adverse response
    d. Developing prodrugs that require enzymatic activation

69. Which of the following is associated with a high risk of opioid overdose?
    a. Daily dose >100 morphine milligram equivalents
    b. Combination of opioids with benzodiazepines
    c. Long-term opioid use (>3 months)
    d. Period >3 months after initiation of longacting opioid formulation

70. High fasting blood cortisol level does not indicate which of the following?
    a. Loss of diurnal variation
    b. Opioid overuse
    c. Adrenal tumor
    d. Exercising

71. Which of the following options is incorrect about the naloxone challenge test?
    a. Assesses lack of physical opioid dependence
    b. Naloxone can be administered via intravenous, subcutaneous, or intramuscular routes
    c. 0.8 mg of naloxone is administered
    d. A negative test guarantees against precipitated opioid withdrawal upon naltrexone administration

72. Weight gain is a side effect of the use of:
    a. Methadone
    b. Buprenorphine
    c. Naltrexone
    d. Clonazepam

73. Lin Zexu's dismantling of the opium trade in Guangdong, China, is commemorated as:
    a. Earth day
    b. International day against drug abuse and illicit trafficking
    c. International opium day
    d. World health day

74. The correct order (from most to least) of the extent of harm caused by drugs is:
    a. Heroin > Cocaine > Cannabis > LSD (lysergic acid diethylamide)
    b. Cocaine > Heroin > Cannabis > Amphetamine
    c. Cocaine > Methamphetamine > LSD > Cannabis
    d. Heroin > Amphetamine > LSD > Cannabis

75. The gene most commonly implicated in the development of opioid addiction is:
    a. ADH1B
    b. OPRM1
    c. ALDH2
    d. CHRM2

76. Chronic opioid use is associated with which of the following phenomena?
    a. Hyperesthesia
    b. Hyperkatifeia
    c. Allodynia
    d. All of the above

77. In animal models, the heroin self-administration was found to be blocked by all, *except*:
    a. Dopamine denervation in the nucleus accumbens
    b. Selective destruction of neurons in the nucleus accumbens
    c. Lesions in the ventral pallidum
    d. Lesions of the pedunculopontine tegmental nucleus

78. Unidirectional cross-tolerance exists between:
    a. Morphine and levorphanol
    b. Morphine and methadone
    c. Morphine and codeine
    d. Morphine and hydrocodone

79. Goldstein's taxonomy of how drugs and crime relate includes all, *except*:
    a. Psychopharmacological
    b. Economic–compulsive
    c. Organic
    d. Systemic

80. Which of the following is a gateway drug according to the gateway drug hypothesis?
    a. Diazepam
    b. Heroin
    c. Alcohol
    d. Codeine

81. Which of the following is a true statement about infective endocarditis in people who inject drugs?
    a. The most common organism is *Pseudomonas* and involves right-side heart valves
    b. The most common organism is *Staphylococcus* and involves right-side heart valves
    c. The most common organism is *Pseudomonas* and involves left-side heart valves
    d. The most common organism is *Staphylococcus* and involves left-side heart valves

82. Complete tolerance among opioids is seen between:
    a. Morphine and codeine
    b. Morphine and morphine-6b-glucuronide
    c. Morphine and heroin
    d. Morphine and methadone

83. Drug not used for maintenance treatment in opioid use disorder is:
    a. Methadone
    b. Heroin
    c. SROM
    d. Carfentanyl

84. The percentage of drug overdose deaths attributed to opioids is:
    a. 70%
    b. 50%
    c. 25%
    d. 10%

85. About the epidemiology of opioid use in India, which of the following statements is incorrect?
    a. The prevalence of current use of any opioid is about 2%
    b. A harmful or dependent pattern is observed in one-fifth of all heroin users compared to half of all opium users
    c. Northeastern states have the highest proportion of population affected by opioid use
    d. Heroin is the most common opioid drug used by people who inject drugs

86. Which of the following drugs does not have mixed agonist and antagonist activity at opioid receptors?
    a. Pentazocine
    b. Butorphanol
    c. Buprenorphine
    d. Levallorphan

87. The duration of the induction phase of maintenance treatment with buprenorphine is usually:
    a. 1 week
    b. 4 weeks
    c. 8 weeks
    d. 12 weeks

88. All are relative contradictions for the use of morphine, *except*:
    a. Hypothyroidism
    b. Multiple sclerosis
    c. Hypervolemic states
    d. Raised biliary tract pressure

89. A patient on buprenorphine maintenance treatment reports taking additional heroin injections, which gives him a feeling of being high. What should be the next step in management?
    a. Stop buprenorphine
    b. Reduce buprenorphine dose to prevent opioid toxicity till he stops injecting
    c. Increase the buprenorphine dose
    d. Switch to methadone

90. All are true about syrup preparation of methadone, *except*:
    a. It has a longer shelf life compared to tablet form
    b. It has a lower abuse potential
    c. It can impair diabetes control
    d. More preferred forms by clients

91. Which of the psychosocial interventions has the least evidence in the management of opioid dependence?
    a. Cognitive behavioral therapy (CBT)
    b. Contingency management
    c. Self-help groups
    d. Insight-oriented psychotherapy

Opioids

92. All are the agents that can decrease methadone levels due to CYP3A4 enzyme interaction, *except*:
    a. Efavirenz
    b. Nevirapine
    c. Amprenavir
    d. Zidovudine

93. Which of the following Indian states has the maximum number of people with opioid-related problems?
    a. Maharashtra
    b. Uttar Pradesh
    c. Punjab
    d. Manipur

94. All are features of NAS, *except*:
    a. Tremors
    b. Hyposensitivity to stimuli
    c. Hypotonia
    d. High-pitched cry

95. All the following statements regarding the pharmacodynamics of opioids are true, *except*:
    a. Pethidine penetrates the blood–brain barrier quicker than morphine
    b. Naloxone is more effective at μ-receptors than at other opioid receptors
    c. Unchanged diamorphine has no affinity for opioid receptors.
    d. Pethidine may be used safely in patients receiving monoamine oxidase inhibitors

96. Regarding partial opioid agonists, all are true, *except*:
    a. Partial agonists are agonists at μ-receptors but antagonists at κ-receptors
    b. Buprenorphine has low intrinsic activity at μ-receptors
    c. Partial agonists show a plateau or ceiling effect in their dose–response curve
    d. Nalbuphine is equipotent to morphine

97. The negative reinforcement theory of opioid dependence postulates a state of .... in the neural system of opioid users, leading to continued use.
    a. Deficit
    b. Allostasis
    c. Hyperexcitability
    d. Instability

98. All are true regarding morphine metabolism, *except*:
    a. The major pathway for elimination is conjugation in the liver with glucuronic acid
    b. The average adult plasma half-life is 2.5–3 hours
    c. Less than 10% is excreted unchanged in the urine in the first 24 hours
    d. Around 50% of the administered dose is excreted in the first 24 hours

99. Which of the following is incorrect regarding neonatal opioid abstinence syndrome?
    a. The onset may be delayed until 7–10 days after birth
    b. Fetal metabolism can determine the severity of symptoms
    c. Heroin-induced symptoms last longer than methadone-induced symptoms
    d. Opioids are a recommended treatment for neonates

100. The creation of a category of "essential narcotic drugs" was a part of:
    a. NDPS Amendments, 1989
    b. NDPS Amendments, 2001
    c. NDPS Amendments, 2014
    d. NDPS Amendments, 2021

101. As per the recent national survey 2019, the number of People Who Inject Drugs in India is:
    a. 8.5 lakh
    b. 15 lakh
    c. 1.5 lakh
    d. 3 lakh

102. A man is caught in possession of 15 g of heroin. What would be the imprisonment in such a case under the NDPS Act?
    a. Up to 1 year of rigorous imprisonment
    b. Up to 10 years of rigorous imprisonment
    c. 10–20 years of rigorous imprisonment
    d. 25 years of imprisonment

103. Which of the following statements is not true about opioid withdrawals?
    a. Diarrhea and abdominal cramps are commonly experienced
    b. Withdrawals of methadone may last for 2–3 weeks
    c. Seizures are commonly seen during opioid withdrawals
    d. Opioid withdrawals are generally not fatal

104. Which of the following drugs is not used to manage opioid withdrawals?
    a. Naltrexone
    b. Buprenorphine
    c. Ibogaine
    d. Dextromethorphan

ANSWER KEY

1. a	2. b	3. a	4. c	5. d	6. d	7. b	8. d
9. a	10. c	11. a	12. d	13. b	14. a	15. a	16. a
17. d	18. c	19. c	20. a	21. d	22. b	23. a	24. d
25. b	26. c	27. a	28. d	29. a	30. c	31. d	32. a
33. a	34. d	35. c	36. a	37. d	38. d	39. a	40. d
41. d	42. a	43. d	44. b	45. a	46. c	47. a	48. c
49. d	50. d	51. a	52. d	53. a	54. c	55. c	56. c
57. a	58. a	59. c	60. b	61. d	62. d	63. c	64. b
65. a	66. b	67. a	68. b	69. d	70. d	71. d	72. a

73. b	74. a	75. b	76. d	77. a	78. a	79. c	80. c
81. b	82. a	83. d	84. a	85. b	86. d	87. a	88. c
89. c	90. d	91. d	92. d	93. b	94. b	95. d	96. a
97. b	98. d	99. c	100. c	101. a	102. b	103. c	104. d

FURTHER READING

1. Brunton L, Hilal-Dandan R, Knollmann BC. Goodman & Gilman's: The Pharmacological Basis of Therapeutics, 13th edition. New York: McGraw Hill; 2017.
2. Karch SB, Drummer O. Karch's Pathology of Drug Abuse, 5th edition. Boca Raton: CRC Press; 2015. p. 912.
3. Kelly JF, Wakeman SE, editors. Treating Opioid Addiction (Current Clinical Psychiatry), 1st edition. Cham: Springer International Publishing; 2019.
4. Koob GF, Arends MA, Le Moal M. Drugs, Addiction, and the Brain, 1st edition. United States: Academic Press; 2014. p. 351.
5. Rao R, Agrawal A, Ambekar A. (2014). Opioid Substitution Therapy under National AIDS Control Programme: Clinical Practice Guidelines for Treatment with Buprenorphine. [online] Available from https://naco.gov.in/sites/default/files/Opiod%20Substitution%20Therapy%20Guideline.pdf [Last accessed November, 2023].
6. Substance Abuse and Mental Health Services Administration. (2021). Medications for Opioid Use Disorder. Treatment Improvement Protocol (TIP) Series 63 Publication No. PEP21-02-01-002. [online] Available from https://store.samhsa.gov/sites/default/files/pep21-02-01-002.pdf [Last accessed November, 2023].

CHAPTER 5

Stimulants, Caffeine, and Inhalants

Siddharth Sarkar, Dhrubajyoti Bhuyan, Manmeet Kaur Brar

1. Which of the following substances do not have the properties of a stimulant?
   a. Betel nut
   b. Mephedrone
   c. Salvinorin A
   d. Methylenedioxymethamphetamine (MDMA)

2. Methamphetamine belongs to which class of compounds?
   a. Phenylethylamine
   b. Piperazine
   c. Pyrrolidine
   d. Imidazole

3. Which of the following is not a cathinone?
   a. Methylone
   b. Methylenedioxypyrovalerone (MDPV)
   c. Spice
   d. Khat

4. What is incorrect about the mechanism of action of methamphetamine?
   a. Methamphetamine act as trace amine-associated receptor 1 (TAAR1) receptor agonist
   b. Methamphetamine acts via sigma and alpha receptors
   c. Methamphetamine acts via inhibiting vesicular monoamine transporter 2 (VMAT2) receptor
   d. Methamphetamines stimulate monoamine oxidase A (MAO-A) and (MAO-B)

5. Which of the following stimulant drugs is not consumed orally?
   a. Ephedra
   b. Yaba
   c. Ice
   d. Crack

6. Which statement is incorrect about the methods and effects of using stimulants?
   a. Concurrent use of cocaine and alcohol is called speedballing
   b. MDMA is commonly used for its entactogenic effects
   c. Doping agencies ban stimulants for their ergogenic effects
   d. Typical cocaine dose when smoked is 50–200 mg

7. What is incorrect about the receptor action of stimulants?
   a. MDMA has a low DAT/SERT (dopamine transporter/serotonin transporter) ratio and is the cause of its entactogenic effects
   b. Cocaine acts as both a transport blocker and transport releaser for catecholamines and serotonin
   c. Amphetamine action as a transport releaser is greater than transport blocker action
   d. L-methamphetamine has more peripheral alpha-adrenergic action than central action

8. Which of the following statements is incorrect?
   a. Cocaine exists as two stereoisomers
   b. Cocaine base has a high melting point and, therefore, is commonly smoked
   c. Cocaine salt is water-soluble and therefore, is commonly injected
   d. Smoking cocaine is more addictive than snorting cocaine

9. What is true about the half-life of stimulants?
   a. $t\frac{1}{2}$ of cocaine is 0.75–1.5 hours
   b. $t\frac{1}{2}$ of methamphetamine is 1.5–2.5 hours
   c. $t\frac{1}{2}$ of amphetamines is 2–4 hours
   d. $t\frac{1}{2}$ of mephedrone is 4–10 hours

10. What is incorrect about the pharmacokinetics of stimulants?
    a. Intranasal stimulants have slower absorption and onset within 30–45 minutes
    b. Inhalation route of stimulant use has rapid absorption and onset of action within 6–8 minutes
    c. Injecting route of stimulant use produced peak brain uptake in 4–7 minutes
    d. Oral route of stimulant use has an onset of action within 60–120 minutes

11. Which statement is incorrect about managing myocardial infarction (MI) due to stimulant use?
    a. Chest pain is typical and similar to pain in MI due to coronary artery disease
    b. Serum troponin is more specific than electrocardiogram (ECG) to make a diagnosis of acute MI due to stimulant use
    c. Benzodiazepines are first line of treatment for hemodynamic stability
    d. Beta blockers are drugs of choice for managing associated hypertensive crisis

12. Which symptom helps differentiate stimulant overdose from opioid overdose?
    a. Mydriasis
    b. Pupillary reaction
    c. Nausea
    d. Hypotension

13. What is correct about oral complications of stimulant use?
    a. Meth mouth leads to caries which typically progress slowly, unlike other causes of dental caries
    b. Cocaine increases the risk of dental caries by two times
    c. Dry mouth is seen in 50% of MDMA users
    d. Bruxism during intoxication can last up to a week

14. Which drug is usually associated with hyponatremia during intoxication?
    a. MDMA
    b. Cocaine
    c. Methamphetamine
    d. MDPV

15. Which statement below is correct about cocaine use adverse effects?
    a. Cocaine use increases the odds of having a seizure by three times
    b. Cocaine use increases the odds of hemorrhagic stroke by six times
    c. Cocaine use increases the odds of ischemic stroke by two times
    d. Cocaine use increases the odds of having a seizure by two times

16. What is correct about managing agitation and paranoia in a patient presenting to emergency with stimulant intoxication?
    a. ART (acceptance, reassurance, talk down) approach is used to calm the patient
    b. Haloperidol is the drug of choice
    c. Urine alkalinization is recommended to increase amphetamine renal excretion
    d. Physical restraint is recommended to protect the patient from harming self or others

17. What is false about Brompton's cocktail?
    a. It was used for palliative care in cancer pain patients
    b. It is a mixture of cocaine, alcohol, morphine, and chloroform
    c. Its use was discontinued due to high risk of overdose and addiction
    d. It is a mixture of caffeine, alcohol, dextromethorphan, and chloroform

18. Which is a common adulterant in cocaine that leads to cutaneous vasculitis?
    a. Lidocaine
    b. Quinone
    c. Levamisole
    d. Benzene

19. What statement regarding the medical use of stimulants is false?
    a. Dextroamphetamine is approved for the treatment of attention-deficit/hyperactivity disorder (ADHD) for children aged 6 years and above
    b. Armodafinil is Food and Drug Administration (FDA)-approved for use in shift-work sleep disorder
    c. Phentermine and topiramate combination is FDA-approved for obesity treatment
    d. Lisdexamfetamine is FDA-approved for ADHD treatment and as an augmentation agent for depression

20. Which statement is incorrect about the legal status of stimulants?
    a. Modafinil is a schedule IV drug
    b. Cocaine is classified under the Convention on Narcotic Drugs 1961
    c. MDMA is a schedule II drug
    d. Amphetamine-type stimulants are classified under the Convention on Psychotropic Substances, 1971

21. Which of the following statements is incorrect about stimulant use in the MSM (men who have sex with men) community?
    a. Serosorting is a practice to reduce hepatitis C virus (HCV) transmission
    b. Blasting refers to injecting drug use of stimulants in the context of ChemSex
    c. ChemSex refers to using methamphetamine, mephedrone, or GHB to facilitate sexual activity
    d. MSM on ART are more likely to engage in ChemSex than those with negative or unknown status

22. Which of the following is NOT a harm reduction practice for stimulant use?
    a. Remaining hydrated while using stimulants
    b. Using mouthpieces for crack pipes
    c. Nasal douching after snorting stimulants
    d. Getting tested for human immunodeficiency virus (HIV) and HCV

23. Which non-pharmacological interventions have maximum evidence for the treatment of stimulant use disorder?
    a. Motivation enhancement therapy (MET) and cognitive behavioral therapy (CBT)
    b. Contingency management and community reinforcement approach
    c. 12-step program and reward-based interventions
    d. Psychodynamic therapy and 12-step program

24. Disulfiram has been tried in randomized controlled trials (RCTs) as a treatment option for which substances?
    a. Methamphetamine
    b. Cocaine
    c. Amphetamine-type stimulants
    d. Opioids

25. Which drug has shown efficacy evidence for light to moderate methamphetamine users?
    a. Bupropion
    b. Disulfiram
    c. Naltrexone
    d. Methylphenidate

26. What is false about drug testing for cocaine?
    a. A single oral dose of cocaine can yield detectable urine concentrations of cocaine metabolites
    b. Passive exposure to cocaine via skin can lead to positive urine drug tests for cocaine metabolites in laboratory personnel
    c. Metabolites of cocaine are not detectable in fetal umbilical cord blood due to maternal antenatal exposure to cocaine
    d. Cocaine's metabolites can be detected in urine for up to 4 days after the last intake

27. Which of the following is the cocaine metabolite detected in urine drug testing for cocaine use when snorted?
    a. Methylecgonine
    b. Anhydroecgonine
    c. Benzoylecgonine
    d. Norcocaine

28. What is false about the metabolism of cocaine?
    a. CYP3A4 metabolizes it
    b. Cocaine metabolite, norcocaine, is cardiotoxic and responsible for its cardiac adverse effects
    c. Butyrylcholinesterases in the liver and plasma metabolize cocaine
    d. Only 5% of cocaine metabolism happens via demethylation

29. Alcohol is often consumed after cocaine intake. However, it is not advisable as:
    a. It will increase the risk of dehydration
    b. Alcohol will prolong cocaine's effect via the formation of a new metabolite, cocaethylene
    c. Both
    d. None

30. Feature in cocaine-induced psychosis that differentiates it from schizophrenia?
    a. More thought disorder
    b. Less negative symptoms
    c. Less tactile hallucinations
    d. More auditory hallucinations

31. Which of the following is the most common withdrawal symptom of stimulant use?
    a. Sleep disturbance
    b. Weight loss
    c. Paranoia
    d. Hallucinations

32. Which neurotransmitter is primarily responsible for the entactogenic effects of MDMA?
    a. Norepinephrine
    b. Dopamine
    c. Serotonin
    d. Glutamate

33. In which country cultivation of the coca plant is illegal?
    a. Bolivia
    b. Peru
    c. Colombia
    d. Portugal

34. Acute administration of stimulants to rodents has been seen to activate the following genes in the brain, *except*:
    a. CREB
    b. c-fos
    c. c-jun
    d. KCNJ6

35. Which substance has been added under disorder due to substance use in ICD-11 (International Classification of Diseases 11th Revision) that was not part of ICD-10 (International Classification of Diseases 10th Revision)?
    a. Disorders to use of cocaine
    b. Disorders due to the use of synthetic cathinone
    c. Disorders due to use of stimulants
    d. Disorders due to the use of caffeine

36. Which is the most commonly consumed psychoactive substance in the world?
    a. Alcohol
    b. Caffeine
    c. Benzodiazepines
    d. Opioids

37. Caffeine belongs to which class of alkaloids?
    a. Methylxanthines
    b. Isoquinoline
    c. Quinoline
    d. Indole

38. A cup of coffee typically contains how much caffeine?
    a. 100–150 µg
    b. 1–1.5 mg
    c. 10–15 mg
    d. 100–150 mg

39. Caffeine is NOT consumed by humans in which form?
    a. Drinks and beverages
    b. Tablets
    c. Combination medicines
    d. Vials

40. What is the half-life of caffeine in the human body?
    a. 10–30 minutes
    b. 1–3 hours
    c. 3–10 hours
    d. 10–30 hours

41. What is the time to peak concentration for caffeine?
    a. 1–3 minutes
    b. 30–60 minutes
    c. 3–10 hours
    d. 10–30 hours

42. What is the mechanism of action of caffeine?
    a. Increase in intraneuronal cyclic adenosine monophosphate (cAMP) concentrations in neurons with adenosine receptor
    b. Increased cyclic guanosine monophosphate (cGMP) concentration in astrocytes with D2 receptors
    c. Decrease in intraneuronal cAMP concentrations in neurons with adenosine receptor
    d. Decrease in cGMP concentration in astrocytes with D2 receptors

43. Which of the following is correct?
    a. Caffeine readily crosses the blood–brain barrier
    b. Caffeine primarily acts on the serotonergic receptor
    c. Caffeine has a half-life of about 1 hour
    d. Caffeine is most commonly consumed as tablets

44. What amount of caffeine causes unpleasant sensations like anxiety and nervousness?
    a. 30–50 mg
    b. 100–150 mg
    c. 10–15 mg
    d. 300–800 mg

45. Which of the following is not described as a pleasurable effect of caffeine?
    a. Increased well-being
    b. Increased concentration
    c. Decreased motivation to work
    d. Decreased tiredness

46. Which of the following statements is incorrect?
    a. Cigarette smokers consume more caffeine than nonsmokers
    b. Heavy use of alcohol is associated with heavy use of caffeine
    c. Individuals with anxiety disorders report higher use levels of caffeine
    d. Caffeine can potentiate the reinforcing effects of nicotine

47. Which of the following is correct?
    a. Caffeine results in global cerebral vasoconstriction
    b. Caffeine results in increased cerebral blood flow
    c. Caffeine results in no change in cerebral blood flow
    d. Caffeine results in global cerebral vasodilatation

48. Which of the following is NOT a differential diagnosis of caffeine dependence?
    a. Generalized anxiety disorder
    b. ADHD
    c. Sleep disorders
    d. Dysthymia

49. Which of the following is not a feature of caffeine intoxication?
    a. Anxiety
    b. Psychomotor agitation
    c. Somnolence
    d. Irritability

50. Which of the following is unlikely to be present in a person with >1 g of caffeine consumption?
    a. Rambling speech
    b. Cardiac arrhythmias
    c. Trailing phenomenon
    d. Tinnitus

51. Which of the following is NOT a feature of caffeine withdrawal state?
    a. Increased concentration
    b. Anxiety
    c. Headache
    d. Nausea

52. When are the caffeine withdrawal symptoms likely to peak after the last caffeine consumption?
    a. 1–2 hours
    b. 8–12 hours
    c. 12–24 hours
    d. 24–48 hours

53. What percentage of caffeine users experience withdrawal symptoms?
    a. About 3–5%
    b. About 20–30%
    c. About 50–75%
    d. About 90–95%

54. Which of the following is NOT associated with caffeine intake?
    a. Diuresis
    b. Cardiac muscle stimulation
    c. Increased gastric acid secretion
    d. Decreased intestinal peristalsis

55. Which of the following measures should NOT be used for managing caffeine withdrawal?
    a. Short duration of benzodiazepines
    b. Fading schedule of caffeine consumption
    c. Sudden cessation of caffeine consumption
    d. Keeping a food diary

56. What is the rate of caffeine decrement recommended for a fading schedule for caffeine?
    a. 2% every few days
    b. 10% every few days
    c. 20% every few days
    d. 50% every few days

57. The pharmacological action of caffeine is:
    a. Nonselective A1 and A2A adenosine receptor antagonist
    b. Nonselective A1 and A2A adenosine receptor agonist
    c. Selective A1 adenosine receptor agonist
    d. Selective A2A adenosine receptor agonist

58. Which of the following products does NOT contain caffeine?
    a. Coffee
    b. Tea
    c. Guarana
    d. Khat

59. Caffeine levels in a fetus are approximately ____ of the blood levels in the mother.
    a. Same
    b. Half
    c. One-third
    d. One-fourth

60. Saliva caffeine levels and plasma caffeine levels have the following relationship:
    a. Significant positive correlation
    b. Significant negative correlation
    c. No correlation
    d. Variable correlation based on the amount of consumption

61. Which of the following is the primary route of metabolism of caffeine?
    a. Cytochrome P-450 liver enzyme system (primarily CYP1A2)
    b. Cytochrome P-450 liver enzyme system (primarily CYP2D6)
    c. Cytochrome P-450 liver enzyme system (primarily CYP2E1)
    d. Largely excreted through the kidneys unmetabolized

62. Which of the following is incorrect?
    a. Consumption of coffee can result in a 10–15 mm increase in systolic blood pressure
    b. Consumption of coffee can result in a 10–15 mm decrease in diastolic blood pressure
    c. Consumption of coffee can increase low-density lipoprotein (LDL) cholesterol
    d. Consumption of coffee can increase total cholesterol

63. Which of the following statements is incorrect?
    a. There is a relationship between caffeine consumption and the likelihood of spontaneous abortion
    b. High caffeine consumption has been associated with reduced fetal growth
    c. High caffeine consumption has been associated with placenta previa
    d. High caffeine consumption has been associated with neural tube defects

64. Which of the following statements is incorrect?
    a. Caffeine increases detrusor instability in patients with this condition
    b. Chronic caffeine consumption can contribute to urinary incontinence in the geriatric population
    c. Reduction of caffeine consumption can improve urinary incontinence
    d. Caffeine consumption can result in urinary retention

Stimulants, Caffeine, and Inhalants

65. Which of the effects of caffeine on exercise is incorrect?
    a. Caffeine can decrease performance during endurance exercise
    b. Caffeine can decrease ratings of perceived exhaustion or effort
    c. Caffeine can improve speed in simulated race conditions
    d. Caffeine can improve power output in simulated race conditions

66. Which of the following statements is incorrect?
    a. Caffeine withdrawal may occur when caffeine users are asked to be nil per oral before surgery
    b. Caffeine withdrawal may cause postoperative headache
    c. Caffeine supplements during surgery may prevent withdrawal
    d. Caffeine use can result in cerebral vasodilation during neurosurgery

67. Which of the following is incorrect regarding the reinforcing effects of caffeine?
    a. Subjects choose caffeine over placebo in double-blind conditions
    b. Doses as low as 25 mg of caffeine are reinforcing
    c. Doses of 100–200 mg/day of caffeine limited to once a day are seen to be reinforcing
    d. Doses of 400 mg or more have higher reinforcing properties of caffeine than 200 mg

68. Caffeine's effect on sleep is:
    a. Wakefulness-promoting, dose-dependent
    b. Wakefulness-promoting, non-dose-dependent
    c. Wakefulness neutral, dose-dependent
    d. Wakefulness neutral, non-dose-dependent

69. Which of the following conditions is recognized in DSM5?
    a. Caffeine-induced sleep disorder
    b. Caffeine-induced sexual dysfunction
    c. Caffeine-induced mood disorder
    d. Caffeine-induced psychotic disorder

70. Which medications can ameliorate the headache associated with caffeine withdrawal?
    a. Analgesic like aspirin
    b. Benzodiazepines like clonazepam
    c. Antidepressants with sedative properties like trazodone
    d. Antipsychotics with sedative properties like quetiapine

71. Woodworking adhesive is a substance mostly abused by people who indulge in abusing volatile substances. Which of the following is the major volatile component in woodworking adhesives?
    a. Butane
    b. Xylenes
    c. Isobutane
    d. Toluenes

72. Which of the following is not a component of cigarette lighter refills?
    a. Butane
    b. Isobutane
    c. Propane
    d. Gasoline

73. Adolescents prefer volatile substances as part of their group activity because of various reasons. Which of the following statements in this regard is incorrect?
    a. These can easily be concealed, or their possession can appear legitimate
    b. The onset of action and recovery is rapid
    c. Less expensive
    d. These can be injected

74. Sudden death is a major risk associated with volatile substance use. Which of the following statements is correct in this regard?
    a. It is often unnoticed and underreported
    b. Trauma, aspiration of vomitus, and asphyxia are identified as the causes of death
    c. Anoxia, respiratory depression, arrhythmia, and sudden cardiac death are the causes of death directly related to volatile substance abuse
    d. All of the above

75. Arrhythmias encountered in individuals using volatile substances are due to:
    a. Vagal stimulation
    b. Sensitization of the heart to circulating catecholamines
    c. All of the above
    d. None of the above

76. Volatile substances, when used, produce effects similar to:
    a. That of opioids and opiates
    b. That of alcohol
    c. That of caffeine
    d. That of cannabis

77. Huffing is a technique of administration of volatile substances in which:
    a. Vapors are directly inhaled from the container
    b. Vapors are inhaled from a cloth soaked in the substance of abuse
    c. Vapors are inhaled from a plastic bag filled with the substance
    d. None of the above

78. The main chemical component of volatile glues, thinners, and aerosol paints responsible for toxicity is:
    a. Toluene
    b. Butane
    c. Gasoline
    d. Ammonia

Stimulants, Caffeine, and Inhalants

79. Which of the following statements is not correct?
    a. Family history of alcohol dependence is a risk factor for volatile substance misuse
    b. There is a high incidence of ADHD, antisocial personality disorder, and poor self-esteem in individuals with volatile substance misuse
    c. Most children experimenting with volatile substances eventually become dependent on them during adulthood
    d. Volatile substance is more common among homeless children

80. Hydrocarbons present in volatile substances act on the brain as:
    a. Stimulants
    b. Depressant
    c. No effect on the brain
    d. None of the above

81. Substituting unleaded petrol with opal is a classic example of:
    a. Harm reduction
    b. Demand reduction
    c. Supply reduction
    d. None of the above

82. Which of the following statements regarding volatile substance intoxication is not correct?
    a. Slowing of thought and perception of time passing very fast is a feature of volatile substances containing toluene
    b. Intoxication can last up to 48 hours
    c. Delusions and hallucinations
    d. Color perception is distorted

83. Which of the following statements is not correct as regards volatile substance withdrawal?
    a. Withdrawal symptoms typically develop within 24–48 hours of cessation
    b. Sleep disturbances, irritability, illusions, tremors, and nausea are typically seen
    c. Stomach cramps, lower chest pain, and tic are commonly reported symptoms
    d. Elated mood

84. Central nervous system (CNS) effects of inhalants are mediated by:
    a. Activation of norepinephrine
    b. Activation of dopamine
    c. Activation of gamma-aminobutyric acid (GABA)
    d. All of the above

85. Which of the following is not a sign of volatile substance abuse?
    a. Huffer rash
    b. Typical odor on body or cloth
    c. Redness of eyes
    d. Hallopeau sign

86. Which of the following statements regarding the mode of administration of volatile substance is correct?
    a. Concentration of substance inhaled from huffing is lower than that from sniffing
    b. Huffing delivers the lowest concentration of the substance
    c. Bagging carries the highest risk of intoxication due to the reuse of the exhaled air
    d. None of the above

87. Choose the correct answer related to CNS complications of volatile substance use.
    a. Decrease the volume of the thalamus
    b. Callosal thinning
    c. Gray matter loss in white matter boundaries
    d. All of the above

88. Volatile substance use can lead to:
    a. Deficit in information processing speed
    b. Impaired working memory
    c. Impaired visual learning
    d. All of the above

89. Which of the following statements is not correct?
    a. Volatile substance use can lead to distal renal acidosis
    b. Volatile substance use can lead to metabolic acidosis with a high anion gap
    c. Volatile substance use disorder can lead to metabolic alkalosis
    d. Volatile substance use can lead to hepatorenal failure

90. Choose the correct answer related to the pulmonary functions in people with volatile substance use.
    a. Increased residual volume
    b. High forced expiratory volume in 1 second (FEV_1)
    c. Increased forced vital capacity (FVC)
    d. None of the above

91. According to the U.S. Occupational Health and Safety Administration (OSHA), the safe limit allowable for toluene is:
    a. 200 ppm
    b. 100 ppm
    c. 500 ppm
    d. 1,000 ppm

92. Which of the following is not a feature of fetal solvent syndrome?
    a. Growth retardation
    b. Macrocephaly
    c. Spatulate fingertips and small fingernails
    d. Micrognathia

93. Which of the following is not a withdrawal symptom of gasoline?
    a. Lacrimation
    b. Salivation
    c. Anhedonia
    d. Psychomotor retardation

94. Which of the following is not true in managing volatile substance intoxication?
    a. Sympathomimetics are to be avoided
    b. Decontamination of skin and clothes
    c. Beta blockers are to be avoided
    d. There is no antidote

95. Primary urinary metabolite of toluene is:
    a. Homovanillic acid
    b. Benzyl benzoate
    c. Hippuric acid
    d. Acetone

96. Which of the following tests is regarded as specific to toluene intoxication?
    a. Urinary hippuric acid
    b. Urinary creatinine level
    c. Ratio of hippuric acid and creatinine in urine
    d. Ratio of Benzoic acid and hippuric acid in urine

97. Which of the following is not an effect of nitrites?
    a. Enhanced sexual feelings
    b. Penile engorgement
    c. Anal sphincter relaxation
    d. Premature ejaculation

98. Butane belongs to which class of chemicals?
    a. Aliphatic hydrocarbons
    b. Aromatic hydrocarbons
    c. Chlorinated hydrocarbons
    d. Esters

99. Which of the following chemicals is popularly known as poppers?
    a. Nitrites
    b. Toluene
    c. Butane
    d. Nitrous oxide

100. Choose the correct statement regarding the mechanism of action of nitrous oxide.
    a. It inhibits glutamate (NMDA) receptors
    b. It activates nicotinic acetylcholine receptors
    c. It inhibits the release of endogenous opioids
    d. All of the above

101. Which of the following is not a feature of benzene toxicity?
   a. Chemical pneumonitis
   b. Hepatorenal syndrome
   c. Aplastic anemia
   d. Pancreatitis

102. Which of the following is not an effect of nitrous oxide?
   a. Decrease in renal blood flow
   b. Increase in hepatic blood flow
   c. Activates chemoreceptor trigger zone
   d. Decreases proprioception

103. Which of the following statements regarding nitrites is true?
   a. It causes intense euphoria
   b. It enhances sexual pleasure
   c. The effect usually lasts for 2 hours
   d. It causes vasoconstriction

104. Which of the following is not an aromatic hydrocarbon?
   a. Toluene
   b. Benzene
   c. Xylene
   d. Propane

105. Which of the following statements regarding toluene is not correct?
   a. It causes activation of the glycine receptor
   b. It suppresses glutamate receptors
   c. It activates nicotinic acetylcholine receptors
   d. It activates serotonin type 3 receptors

ANSWER KEY

1. c	2. a	3. c	4. d	5. d	6. a	7. b	8. b
9. a	10. d	11. d	12. a	13. a	14. a	15. c	16. a
17. d	18. c	19. d	20. c	21. a	22. d	23. b	24. b
25. a	26. c	27. c	28. b	29. c	30. b	31. a	32. c
33. d	34. d	35. b	36. b	37. a	38. d	39. d	40. c
41. b	42. a	43. a	44. d	45. c	46. c	47. a	48. d
49. c	50. c	51. a	52. d	53. c	54. d	55. c	56. b
57. a	58. d	59. a	60. a	61. a	62. b	63. c	64. d
65. a	66. d	67. d	68. a	69. a	70. a	71. b	72. d
73. d	74. d	75. c	76. b	77. b	78. a	79. c	80. b
81. c	82. b	83. d	84. d	85. d	86. c	87. d	88. d
89. c	90. a	91. a	92. b	93. b	94. c	95. c	96. c
97. d	98. a	99. a	100. a	101. d	102. b	103. b	104. d
105. c							

FURTHER READING

1. Boland RJ, Verduin ML, Ruiz P, Arya Shah, Sadock BJ. Kaplan & Sadock's Synopsis of Psychiatry, 12th edition. Philadelphia: Wolters Kluwer; 2022.
2. Cruz SL, Bowen SE. The last two decades on preclinical and clinical research on inhalant effects. Neurotoxicol Teratol. 2021;87:106999.
3. El-Guebaly N, Carrà G, Galanter M, Baldacchino AM. Textbook of Addiction Treatment. Cham: Springer; 2021.
4. Miller SC, Fiellin DA, Rosenthal RN, Saitz R; American Society Of Addiction Medicine. The ASAM Principles of Addiction Medicine, 6th edition. Philadelphia: Wolters Kluwer; 2019.
5. Ronsley C, Nolan S, Knight R, Hayashi K, Klimas J, Walley A, et al. Treatment of stimulant use disorder: A systematic review of reviews. Hashimoto K, editor. PLoS One. 2020;15(6):e0234809.

CHAPTER 6

Hallucinogens, Phencyclidine, and Methylenedioxymethamphetamine

Arpit Parmar, Amit Singh, Arghya Pal

1. "Yellow Sunshine" and "Blotter Acid" are the street names of which of the following substances?
   a. Phencyclidine [phenylcyclohexyl piperidine (PCP)]
   b. Lysergic acid diethylamide (LSD)
   c. Dimethyltryptamine (DMT)
   d. Psilocybin

2. The magic mushrooms often consumed for hallucinogenic effects are indigenous to which region?
   a. Latin and Central America
   b. Asia
   c. Africa
   d. Oceania

3. The deliriant group of hallucinogens acts through which receptors?
   a. Serotonergic receptors
   b. Cannabinoid receptors
   c. Cholinergic receptors
   d. Dopaminergic receptors

4. The effects of the dissociative anesthetist are mediated through which receptors?
   a. Serotonergic receptors
   b. Cannabinoid receptors
   c. N-methyl-D-aspartate (NMDA) receptors
   d. Dopaminergic receptors

5. "Angel Dust" and "Peace Pill" are the street names of which of the following substances?
   a. Phencyclidine
   b. LSD
   c. DMT (LSD)
   d. Psilocybin

6. Which of the following statements can be considered false for hallucinogens?
   a. Research has shown that using hallucinogens as the primary substance is relatively rare
   b. Hallucinogen use can lead to a higher predisposition to develop psychotic disorders
   c. Lifetime use of hallucinogens was related to a lower occurrence of post-traumatic stress disorder (PTSD)
   d. Lifetime use of hallucinogens was associated with significantly higher co-occurrence of alcohol use disorder

7. Which of the following conditions is the most common reason for clinical contact following hallucinogen use?
   a. Hallucinogen use disorder
   b. Hallucinogen intoxication
   c. Hallucinogen withdrawal
   d. Hallucinogen-persisting perception disorder (HPPD)

8. Which of the following types of hallucinogen potentially has the longest duration of psychotropic effects?
   a. Phencyclidine
   b. LSD
   c. DMT
   d. Psilocybin

9. Which of the following is uncommon when using LSD?
   a. Marcus Gunn pupil
   b. Mydriasis
   c. Anisocoria
   d. Hippus

10. Which of the following statements regarding HPPD type I is untrue?
    a. It has a chronic and protracted course
    b. It is usually benign
    c. It is associated with minimal dysfunction
    d. Patients appreciate it as free trips as they enable them to relive the intoxicating effects of the hallucinogens

11. Which of the following entities is not a recognized diagnosis according to DSM 5 (Diagnostic and Statistical Manual of Mental Disorders, 5th edition)?
    a. Hallucinogen use disorder
    b. Hallucinogen intoxication
    c. Hallucinogen withdrawal
    d. HPPD

12. The diagnostic criteria for which of the following substances has 10 items to be diagnosed as "use disorder" as opposed to the traditional 11 items according to DSM 5?
    a. Alcohol
    b. Opioid
    c. Tobacco
    d. Phencyclidine (PCP)

13. Which of the following hallucinogens is considered to have a very low abuse potential and thus rarely causes the development of tolerance?
    a. Mescaline
    b. DMT
    c. LSD
    d. Phencyclidine

14. Which of the following hallucinogens is most used through the parenteral route?
    a. Ketamine
    b. LSD
    c. DMT
    d. NBOMe

15. Who is credited with the discovery of LSD?
    a. Albert Hofmann
    b. Timothy Leary
    c. Maria Sabina
    d. Alexander Shulgin

16. The works of Maria Sabina, a Mexican Poet, were deemed to be heavily influenced by the effects of which hallucinogen?
    a. Mescaline
    b. Psilocybin
    c. LSD
    d. Phencyclidine

17. Which of the following has NOT been tried as a therapeutic effect of LSD?
    a. Alcohol dependence
    b. Police interrogation
    c. Spiritual practices
    d. Panic disorder

18. LSD was derived initially from which fungus?
    a. Psilocybin
    b. Ergot
    c. Cordyceps
    d. Agaricus

19. Which of the following hallucinogens is classified as a deliriant?
    a. Datura
    b. Ibogaine
    c. Mescaline
    d. Cannabis

20. Which of the following is not a recognized sign of hallucinogen intoxication?
    a. Tremors
    b. Bradycardia
    c. Sweating
    d. Blurring of vision

21. Which of the following agents is also considered a stimulant and a hallucinogen?
    a. Atropine
    b. 3,4-Methylenedioxymethamphetamine (MDMA)
    c. Mescaline
    d. Phencyclidine (PCP)

22. Which of the following is not traditionally considered a subtype of hallucinogen?
    a. Stimulants
    b. Deliriants
    c. Entactogens
    d. Psychedelics

23. Which of the following is not a tool to study mystical experiences?
    a. Hood's Mysticism Scale
    b. Spiritual Transcendence Scale
    c. Mystical Experience Questionnaire
    d. Centrality of Religiosity Scale

24. Which of the following methods is not a common mode of using hallucinogens?
    a. Brewing as a tea
    b. Consuming pills

c. Swallowing as soaked objects
d. Huffing

25. Which of the following is not a common co-occurring disorder with hallucinogen use disorder?
    a. Major depressive disorder
    b. Functional neurological symptom disorder
    c. Alcohol use disorder
    d. PTSD

26. A 23-year-old female presents to the emergency department with a history of ingesting LSD at a party. Her friends brought her after she started laughing uncontrollably and started perspiring. In the emergency department, a provisional diagnosis of LSD intoxication was made. Which of the following is not a usual sign of LSD intoxication?
    a. Hypothermia
    b. Tachycardia
    c. Coma
    d. QT prolongation

27. A 22-year-old male is brought to the emergency department after he presented with irrelevant speech, hallucinatory behavior, and anxiety symptoms. His friends report that they brought him because they had witnessed at least two similar presentations during which he became unmanageable and violent and for which the patient required admission. Which of the following measures is least expected to be needed for this patient when the patient is being worked up in emergency?
    a. Access to injectable benzodiazepines
    b. Room heater
    c. Alert security staff
    d. Access to restraints

28. Which of the following statements regarding HPPD type II is untrue?
    a. Stressful situations precipitate it
    b. It has a chronic course
    c. It is associated with significant dysfunction
    d. Patients appreciate it as free trips as they enable them to relive the intoxicating effects of the hallucinogens

29. Special K is a street name for which of the following compounds?
    a. Esketamine
    b. Khat
    c. Ketamine
    d. Krokodil

30. Which of the following hallucinogens is classified as an entactogen?
    a. 3,4-MDMA
    b. DMT
    c. LSD
    d. Ibogaine

31. As per the recent national drug survey of India (2019), what is the prevalence of hallucinogen use in the past 12 months in India?
    a. 0.85%
    b. 1.5%
    c. 0.12%
    d. 3.1%

32. Which of the following states has the highest number of hallucinogen users in India?
    a. Maharashtra
    b. Telangana
    c. Goa
    d. Kerala

33. As per the Narcotic Drugs and Psychotropics Substances Act, 1985, what is the commercial quantity of MDMA (Ecstasy)?
    a. 5 g
    b. 0.5 g
    c. 20 g
    d. 10 g

34. Acute LSD intoxication may last for up to …
    a. 12 hours
    b. 24 hours
    c. 36 hours
    d. 4 hours

35. Mr. A consumed a pill orally for the first time. After about 1 hour, he reports experiencing feeling closeness to others, increased empathy, and increased sociability. Which of the following drugs he might have consumed?
    a. MDMA (3,4-methylenedioxy-N-methylamphetamine)
    b. Ketamine
    c. LSD
    d. Phencyclidine (PCP)

36. All of the following drugs' intoxication may cause piloerection, *except*:
    a. Opioids
    b. LSD
    c. 3,4-MDMA
    d. Phencyclidine (PCP)

37. In contrast to other drugs, one of the following hallucinogenic drugs is associated with dysphoria, sadness, and depression.
    a. LSD
    b. Ibogaine
    c. Mescaline
    d. Salvinorin A

38. Which receptor is considered the primary target for all serotonergic hallucinogens (such as LSD, psilocybin, and mescaline)?
    a. 5-HT2_A
    b. 5-HT2_B
    c. 5-HT2_C
    d. 5-HT2_D

39. What is the proportion of people who develop hallucinogen use disorder following hallucinogen use ever?
    a. 10.5%
    b. 0.65%
    c. 3.4%
    d. 15%

40. All of the following factors contribute to the low-addiction liability of hallucinogens, *except*:
    a. Hallucinogens are not consistently reinforcing in terms of positive reinforcement
    b. Rapid tolerance to the rewarding effects
    c. Absence of withdrawal symptoms
    d. Absence of intoxication

41. Which of the following statements about LSD is incorrect?
    a. LSD can be administered only by oral route
    b. LSD has psychoactive effects at a dose as low as 20 µg
    c. Levels of LSD peak at around 1.5 hours after the administration
    d. LSD may induce mydriasis, tachycardia, nausea, and vomiting

42. All of the following statements about the subjective and psychological effects of LSD are true, *except*:
    a. The effects last for up to 10 hours
    b. LSD may cause depersonalization and derealization
    c. Insight is usually absent
    d. It does not cause persistent cognitive impairment

43. All of the following drugs are indoleamides, *except*:
    a. LSD
    b. Psilocybin
    c. Ibogaine
    d. Mescaline

44. Which of the following substances is known to enhance music-evoked emotion?
    a. Cannabis
    b. Opioids
    c. LSD
    d. Amphetamine

45. In 2020, the Food and Drug Administration (FDA)-approved the following drug for the management of treatment-resistant depression:
    a. Oral ketamine
    b. Intravenous (IV) ketamine
    c. Oral ketamine
    d. Intranasal esketamine

46. Ayahuasca contains all of the following, *except*:
    a. DMT
    b. Harmine
    c. Harmaline
    d. Phencyclidine

47. Tolerance does not develop rapidly in humans for one of the following hallucinogens:
    a. LSD
    b. Psilocybin
    c. Mescaline
    d. DMT

48. The somatic effects of 3,4-MDMA include all of the following, *except*:
    a. Increased appetite
    b. Diaphoresis
    c. Mydriasis
    d. Bruxism

49. Which of the following statements about the pharmacology of 3,4-MDMA is correct?
    a. It increases blood pressure in a dose-dependent manner
    b. The effects last for 24 hours
    c. MDMA is a potent 5-HT2A agonist
    d. Acute MDMA use does not alter cortisol and prolactin levels

50. All of the following features characterize hallucinogen-associated psychosis, *except*:
    a. All kinds of hallucinations may occur
    b. "Talking down" the patient is the most common way to ease the anxiety
    c. The psychiatric diagnosis most commonly associated with post-LSD psychosis is a form of schizoaffective disorder
    d. Most common hallucinations are auditory

51. Which of the following molecules is also known as the "businessman's LSD"?
    a. Psilocybin
    b. Mescaline
    c. DMT
    d. 3,4-MDMA

52. What is not true for the tolerance of hallucinogens?
    a. A high degree of tolerance develops for the effects of LSD after repeated administration
    b. Tolerance is lost rapidly after one ceases using LSD for several days
    c. Cross-tolerance develops between LSD and other drugs such as phencyclidine, marihuana, and 3,4-MDMA
    d. Little tolerance develops to the autonomic effects of hallucinogens

53. Which of the following is not reported as an acute complication of LSD use?
    a. Posterior reversible encephalopathy
    b. Seizures
    c. Serotonin syndrome
    d. Psychosis

54. Which drugs are approved for treating flashbacks associated with using LSD?
    a. Risperidone
    b. Tricyclic antidepressants (TCAs)
    c. Selective serotonin reuptake inhibitors (SSRIs)
    d. None of the above

55. Which of the following drugs is commonly referred to as a "designer drug"?
    a. LSD
    b. PCP
    c. Mescaline
    d. DMT

56. Which of the following drugs is commonly used as an adulterant with other illicit substances?
    a. PCP
    b. Cocaine
    c. Ketamine
    d. LSD

57. Features of 3,4-MDMA toxicity include all the following, *except*:
    a. Rhabdomyolysis
    b. Acute hyperthermia
    c. Hypernatremia
    d. Cerebral edema

58. The act of smoking crack cocaine with phencyclidine (PCP) is known as:
    a. Speedballing
    b. Primos
    c. Space basing
    d. Brompton cocktail

59. Which symptoms are not included in the DSM-5 diagnostic criteria of phencyclidine (PCP) intoxication?
    a. Nystagmus
    b. Hyperacusis
    c. Bradycardia
    d. Numbness

60. Which of the following pairs about drugs and their street names must be corrected?
    a. 3,4-MDMA—Ecstasy
    b. 3,4-Methylenedioxyamphetamine (MDA)—Love pill
    c. 3,4-Methylenedioxyethylamphetamine (MDEA)—Eve
    d. DMT—Acid

61. Peyote is a cactus found in the Southwestern USA and Mexico. Native people used this plant to produce visions. What is the name of the psychoactive alkaloid that is derived from this plant?
    a. Mescaline
    b. Psilocybin
    c. Psilocin
    d. Ibogaine

62. Mescaline, 3,4-MDMA, LSD, and psilocybin are included in which schedule of the United Nations Convention on Psychotropic Substances 1971?
    a. Schedule 1
    b. Schedule 2
    c. Schedule 3
    d. Schedule 4

63. Which of the following drugs was granted the "Breakthrough Therapy" designation by the US FDA for the treatment of PTSD in 2017?
    a. LSD
    b. 3,4-MDMA
    c. DMT
    d. 5-MeO-DMT

64. Which drug has been approved recently for prescription by psychiatrists in resistant mental illnesses such as depression in Australia?
   a. LSD
   b. DMT
   c. Psilocybin
   d. Khat

65. As per the World Drug Report 2023, what is the past-year prevalence of 3,4-MDMA use globally?
   a. 1%
   b. 0.4%
   c. 1.7%
   d. 0.02%

66. Which of the following statements regarding flashbacks associated with hallucinogens is false?
   a. It can be precipitated by sexual intercourse, exercise, or pregnancy
   b. Up to 60% of LSD users experience flashbacks
   c. The frequency of flashbacks increases with time
   d. The most common flashback phenomena are visual

67. Mark the correct statement about managing hallucinogen use disorder treatment.
   a. No specific drugs have been approved to treat this disorder
   b. "Bad trip" generally required admission in the inpatient setup
   c. The best choice of drug in acute cases is atypical antipsychotics
   d. "Bad trip" is associated with permanent cognitive damage

68. Psilocybin is converted in the body into _____, a pharmacologically active compound.
   a. Psilocin
   b. PMA (paramethoxyamphetamine)
   c. LSD
   d. MBDB (N-methyl-1-(1,3-benzodioxol-5-yl)-2-aminobutanamine)

69. All of the following statements about dextromethorphan (DXM) are true, *except*:
   a. It is commonly used as a cough suppressant
   b. It is used as an adjunct to morphine in pain treatment
   c. Naloxone can be used as a specific antidote in case of toxicity
   d. It acts by NMDA glutamate receptor antagonism

70. Choose the correct statement about salvinorin A.
   a. It is one of the most potent naturally occurring hallucinogens
   b. It acts as a selective kappa opioid receptor antagonist
   c. It is a potent D2 partial agonist
   d. The action lasts for around 30 minutes

71. Which of the following is not a mechanism of action of ibogaine?
    a. 5-HT2A receptor agonist
    b. NMDA antagonist
    c. Opioid kappa receptor agonist
    d. Opioid μ-receptor partial agonist

72. All of the following are plant-based hallucinogens, *except*:
    a. Ibogaine
    b. Psilocybin
    c. Mescaline
    d. Phencyclidine (PCP)

73. The Indian Police arrested an individual with 1 g of LSD. What would be the punishment for this crime under the NDPS Act, 1985?
    a. Up to 1 year
    b. 1–10 years
    c. 10–20 years
    d. 5–10 years

74. All of the following are classic hallucinogens, *except*:
    a. LSD
    b. DMT
    c. Salvinorin A
    d. Mescaline

75. Which of the following statements about psychedelic therapy is false?
    a. High doses of LSD are used
    b. The goal is one to three "overwhelming experiences"
    c. Adaption to reality is the main purpose
    d. It is potentially useful in alcoholism and terminal cancer patients

76. Which of the following therapy aims to provide direct satisfaction for physical affection by providing close physical contact during sessions?
    a. Anaclitic therapy
    b. Psycholytic therapy
    c. Psychedelic therapy
    d. Hypnodelic therapy

77. Who coined the term *psychedelic*?
    a. Aldous Huxley
    b. Humphry Osmond
    c. Albert Hoffman
    d. Sigmund Freud

78. Which of the following hallucinogens is associated with QT prolongation?
    a. LSD
    b. Phencyclidine (PCP)
    c. Mescaline
    d. Ibogaine

79. Which of the following statements about the "bad trip" of LSD is untrue?
    a. It is characterized by paranoia, anxiety, dysphoria, panic, agitation, and fear of losing one's mind
    b. It is more common among those with a trauma or mental illness history
    c. Users retain insight during such episodes
    d. It generally does not occur in recreational settings

80. All of the following are potential risk factors for HPPD, *except*:
    a. Recent onset of hallucinogen use
    b. Comorbid cannabis use
    c. Comorbid alcohol use
    d. Comorbid panic disorder

81. Mark the false statement about mescaline.
    a. Mescaline effects last for 6–8 hours
    b. Mescaline easily passes the blood–brain barrier
    c. Arthur Heffer isolated mescaline from peyote cactus for the first time
    d. It works primarily on 5-HT2$_A$

82. Which of the following classic psychedelics regarding chemical structure differs from the other three?
    a. LSD
    b. Psilocybin
    c. DMT
    d. Mescaline

83. Which hallucinogens are used for acute withdrawal management in opioid use disorder?
    a. LSD
    b. 3,4-MDMA
    c. Ibogaine
    d. Phencyclidine (PCP)

84. Ecstacy is a street name for which hallucinogen?
    a. LSD
    b. Phencyclidine (PCP)
    c. 3,4-MDMA
    d. Ibogaine

85. Zombie-like ataxic gait or "zombie walk" has been reported with an overdose of which drugs?
    a. DXM
    b. LSD
    c. Phencyclidine (PCP)
    d. Mescaline

86. Which of the following statements is incorrect for 3,4-MDMA detection in body fluids?
    a. MDMA concentrations in the oral fluid are affected by pH
    b. MDMA can be detected in sweat for 2–12 hours after ingestion
    c. There is no relation between administered dose and concentration in oral fluid
    d. MDA, the metabolite of MDMA, has a role in the neurotoxicity of MDMA

87. Which of the following hallucinogens has not been included under the psychotropics list of the NDPS Act, 1985?
    a. LSD
    b. Salvinorin A
    c. Mescaline
    d. Phencyclidine

88. "Going pharming" or "robodosing" are terms used for the recreational use of which of the following substances?
    a. LSD
    b. Ketamine
    c. DXM
    d. Phencyclidine (PCP)

89. Which of the following statements about DXM use is incorrect?
    a. It is a D-isomer of codeine synthetic analog
    b. DXM may cause complete dissociation with unresponsiveness at a dose of 2.5–7.5 mg/kg
    c. DXM may cause serotonin syndrome, especially when co-ingested with SSRIs
    d. Hallucinations are caused by the effect of dextrorphan, an active metabolite that inhibits NMDA receptors

90. Mark the incorrect statement about salvinorin A.
    a. Plant Salvia divinorum is endemic to southern Mexico
    b. Traditionally, the leaves of the plants are used as an aqueous infusion or as a chewed quid
    c. Salvinorin A has high selectivity and efficacy for kappa opioid receptors
    d. Inhaled salvinorin A has a long duration of action

91. "Bicycle day" is associated with which psychoactive substance?
    a. Cannabis
    b. Opioids
    c. LSD
    d. Amphetamine

92. "Good Friday experiment" involved the use of which of the following substance?
    a. Psilocybin
    b. Cannabis
    c. LSD
    d. Amphetamine

93. Which of the following has no anesthetic properties?
    a. S. divinorum
    b. Phencyclidine (PCP)
    c. Ketamine
    d. Gamma hydroxybutyrate (GHB)

94. The bioavailability of oral ketamine is:
    a. 17%
    b. 42%
    c. 73%
    d. 94%

95. DXM does not act on the following receptor:
    a. NMDA
    b. µ opioid receptor
    c. σ opioid receptor
    d. H1 receptor

96. What percentage of LSD users develop persistent psychosis?
    a. 0.08–4.6%
    b. 6.2–8.5%
    c. 10%
    d. 15–17%

97. K-hole is a phenomenon associated with the psychological effects of one of the following drugs:
    a. Khat
    b. Krokodil
    c. Ketamine
    d. Kratom

98. Which of the following is the most common symptom of HPPD?
    a. Paranoid ideations
    b. Tactile hallucinations
    c. Slow motion phenomenon
    d. Color confusion and geometric hallucinations

99. Mark the wrong statement about mescaline.
    a. It can be taken orally or injected
    b. Psychological symptoms appear first, usually
    c. The entire experience of effects lasts for around 12 hours
    d. Tolerance to its effects develops rapidly

100. Which drug is a selective kappa opioid receptor agonist?
    a. Buprenorphine
    b. Ibogaine
    c. Pentazocine
    d. Salvinorin A

ANSWER KEY

1. b	2. a	3. c	4. c	5. a	6. c	7. b	8. a
9. a	10. a	11. c	12. d	13. b	14. a	15. a	16. b
17. d	18. b	19. a	20. b	21. b	22. a	23. d	24. d
25. b	26. a	27. b	28. d	29. c	30. a	31. c	32. a
33. d	34. a	35. a	36. a	37. d	38. a	39. b	40. d
41. a	42. c	43. d	44. c	45. d	46. d	47. d	48. a
49. a	50. d	51. c	52. c	53. c	54. d	55. b	56. a
57. c	58. c	59. c	60. d	61. a	62. a	63. b	64. c
65. b	66. c	67. a	68. a	69. c	70. b	71. d	72. d
73. c	74. c	75. c	76. a	77. b	78. d	79. d	80. a
81. b	82. d	83. c	84. c	85. a	86. d	87. b	88. c
89. b	90. d	91. c	92. a	93. a	94. a	95. d	96. a
97. c	98. d	99. b	100. d				

FURTHER READING

1. Farré M, Papaseit E, Fonseca F, Torrens M. Addiction of Hallucinogens, Dissociatives, Designer Drugs and "Legal Highs": Update on Potential Therapeutic Use. Textbook of Addiction Treatment: International Perspectives. 2021;259-79.

2. Herron A, Brennan TK. The ASAM essentials of addiction medicine. Lippincott Williams & Wilkins; 2019.
3. Lowinson, JH Lowinson and Ruiz's substance abuse: A comprehensive textbook. Lippincott Williams & Wilkins; 2011.
4. Miller PM. Comprehensive addictive behaviors and disorders. Academic Press/Elsevier; 2015.
5. Miller S. The ASAM principles of addiction medicine. Lippincott Williams & Wilkins; 2018.
6. Preedy VR (Ed.). Neuropathology of Drug Addictions and Substance Misuse Volume 2: Stimulants, Club and Dissociative Drugs, Hallucinogens, Steroids, Inhalants and International Aspects. Academic Press; 2016.

CHAPTER 7

Hypnotics and Prescription Drug Abuse

Sourav Khanra, Aniruddha Mukherjee, Tathagata Mahintamani

1. Which of the following is not a typical pharmacological action of benzodiazepines (BZDs)?
   a. Anticonvulsive
   b. Anxiolytic
   c. Analgesic
   d. Amnestic

2. Which of the following statements is false about gamma-aminobutyric acid type A (GABA-A) receptor?
   a. They conduct chloride ions across neuronal cell membranes
   b. GABA-A receptor has five subunits
   c. There are two GABA-binding sites in the receptor
   d. BZDs bind to the GABA-binding site of the receptor

3. Which of the following belongs to the 2,3-benzodiazepine family?
   a. Clonazepam
   b. Tofisopam
   c. Oxazepam
   d. Nitrazepam

4. Which of the following benzodiazepines has the shortest half-life?
   a. Chlordiazepoxide
   b. Lorazepam
   c. Clonazepam
   d. Diazepam

5. Which of the following is not an equivalent dose of diazepam 5 mg?
   a. Alprazolam 0.5 mg
   b. Estazolam 0.5 mg
   c. Clonazepam 0.5 mg
   d. Triazolam 0.5 mg

6. Which of the following is used to reverse an overdose of benzodiazepine?
   a. Naloxone
   b. Naltrexone
   c. Flumazenil
   d. Dantrolene

7. Which of the following has the shortest half-life?
   a. Zolpidem
   b. Zaleplon
   c. Zopiclone
   d. Eszopiclone

8. Which of the following statements about the effect of benzodiazepines on sleep architecture are correct?
   i. Benzodiazepines increase stage N1 sleep
   ii. Benzodiazepines increase stage N2 sleep
   iii. Benzodiazepines increase slow-wave sleep
   iv. Benzodiazepines increase rapid eye movement (REM) sleep

a. i.—True, ii.—False, iii.—True, iv.—False
   b. i.—False, ii.—True, iii.—True, iv.—False
   c. i.—True, ii.—True, iii.—False, iv.—False
   d. i.—True, ii.—False, iii.—False, iv.—True

9. Which of the following sleep medicine is the least habit-forming?
   a. Alprazolam
   b. Ramelteon
   c. Zolpidem
   d. Lemborexant

10. *Statement A*: Benzodiazepines act on GABA-A receptors.
    Statement B: Benzodiazepines act on GABA-B receptors.
    Which of the statements is true?
    a. Statement A is correct, but B is incorrect
    b. Statement A is incorrect, but B is correct
    c. Both statements are correct
    d. Both statements are incorrect

11. Which of the following is metabolized in the liver by cytochrome P450 system (phase I)?
    a. Lorazepam
    b. Quazepam
    c. Oxazepam
    d. Temazepam

12. Which of the following should be used to treat an overdose of "Z" compound hypnotics?
    a. Dantrolene
    b. Flumazenil
    c. Naltrexone
    d. Buprenorphine

13. Which of the following is not true for Flumazenil?
    a. It has a high affinity to the benzodiazepine-binding site on the GABA-A receptor
    b. It antagonizes the electrophysiological and behavioral effects of benzodiazepines
    c. It antagonizes the electrophysiological and behavioral effects of β-carbolines
    d. A single bolus injection administration is preferred to a series of small injections

14. Which of the following is not true for ramelteon?
    a. Activate melatonin receptors in the suprachiasmatic nuclei
    b. Decrease the latency of sleep onset with minimal rebound insomnia or withdrawal symptoms
    c. Direct effects on GABA-ergic neurotransmission in the central nervous system (CNS)
    d. Adverse effects include dizziness, fatigue, and endocrine changes, including decreased testosterone and increased prolactin

15. Which of the following are naturally occurring alkaloids derived from *Papaver somniferum*?
    a. Papaverine, morphine, codeine, thebaine
    b. Morphine, pethidine, methadone, codeine
    c. Codeine, naloxone, fentanyl, morphine
    d. Buprenorphine, diamorphine, propoxyphene, naloxone

16. Naloxone does not have affinity for which of the following opioid receptors?
    a. δ-opioid receptor
    b. κ-opioid receptor
    c. μ-opioid receptor
    d. Nociceptin orphanin receptor

17. Chronic laxative abuse can lead to all of the following, *except*?
    a. Electrolyte imbalances
    b. Dehydration
    c. Rectal prolapse
    d. None of the above

18. Out of the following, laxative abuse is least likely to be seen in:
    a. Bulimia nervosa
    b. Anorexia nervosa
    c. Mania
    d. Munchausen syndrome

19. Which of the following is not a designer benzodiazepine?
    a. Alprazolam
    b. Clonazolam
    c. Ketazolam
    d. Flutazolam

20. Tramadol has close structural similarities with:
    a. Mirtazapine
    b. Fluoxetine
    c. Venlafaxine
    d. Amitriptyline

21. Deprescribing is relevant for:
    a. Elderly
    b. Anxiolytics
    c. Polypharmacy
    d. All of the above

22. Promiscuous sexual behavior is with:
    a. Temazepam
    b. Flunitrazepam
    c. Oxazepam
    d. None of the above

23. Which of the following statements is true for these drugs? The drugs are: i. chloral hydrate, ii. methaqualone, iii. meprobamate, and iv. ethchlorvynol
    a. All of these are related
    b. Only i. and ii. are related
    c. Only ii. and iii. are related
    d. Only iii. and iv. are related

24. All of the following are true for GABA-A receptors, *except*:
    a. Pentameric
    b. Total 19 subunits
    c. Genes arranged in clusters
    d. Beta has the maximum number of subunits

25. Benzodiazepines binds at:
    a. α+/γ– interface of GABA-A receptor
    b. β+/α– interface of GABA-A receptor
    c. β+/γ– interface of GABA-A receptor
    d. None of the above

26. Benzodiazepine-sensitive GABA-A receptors have the following structure configuration?
    a. One α subunit with two β subunits and a γ subunit
    b. Two α subunits with one β subunit and a γ subunit
    c. Two α subunits with two β subunits and a γ subunit
    d. Two α subunits with two β subunits and two γ subunits

27. Which GABA-A receptor subunit is exclusively extrasynaptically located?
    a. Alpha
    b. Beta
    c. Gamma
    d. Delta

28. Which of the following is false for orthosteric agonists?
    a. They bind to GABA-binding site
    b. Gabazine is not an example
    c. Effects conformational changes in the receptor
    d. Increase chloride conductance

29. GABA-A receptors having the ability of only tonic inhibition must have:
    a. Alpha subunit
    b. Beta subunit
    c. Delta subunit
    d. Epsilon subunit

30. Which of the following is not mentioned in the abuse of non-dependence-producing substances section of ICD-10 (International Classification of Diseases 10th Revision)?
    a. Statins
    b. Diuretics
    c. Vitamins
    d. Hormones

31. Which of the following is present in Syrup Corex T?
    a. Codeine
    b. Dextromethorphan
    c. Hydrocodone
    d. Oxycodone

32. All of the following is present in tablet Spasmo Proxyvon, *except*?
    a. Dicyclomine
    b. Paracetamol
    c. Tramadol
    d. Ibuprofen

33. Which of the following schedules of the Drugs and Cosmetic Act, 1945 deals with prescription drugs?
    a. J
    b. H
    c. X
    d. G

34. Which of the following schedules of the Drugs and Cosmetic Act, 1945 deals with diseases for which drugs may not purport to prevent or cure or make claims to prevent or cure?
    a. J
    b. H
    c. X
    d. G

35. Which of the following schedules enlist drugs for which the retailer must retain a copy of the prescription?
    a. J
    b. H
    c. X
    d. G

36. The following are prescription drugs as mentioned in the Drug and Cosmetics Act, 1945, *except*:
    a. Pentobarbital
    b. Pentoxifylline
    c. Polidocanol
    d. Propofol

37. Benzodiazepines affect:
    a. Short-term memory
    b. Sensory memory
    c. Episodic memory
    d. Semantic memory

38. A "differential time course" patterned benzodiazepine-induced effect is seen in:
    a. Short-term memory
    b. Sensory memory
    c. Implicit memory
    d. Explicit memory

39. Which of the following is an incorrect match?
    a. Sedative—Moderates excitement
    b. Hypnotic—Facilitates maintenance of sleep
    c. Sedative—Decreases activity
    d. Hypnotic—The recipient cannot be aroused easily

40. Abrupt stopping of long-term high-dose benzodiazepine use can lead to:
    a. Seizures
    b. Delirium
    c. Both of the above
    d. None of the above

41. Which among the following is the longest-acting benzodiazepine or related drug?
    a. Flurazepam
    b. Triazolam
    c. Zolpidem
    d. Temazepam

42. A benzodiazepine should be tapered rather than discontinued abruptly if it has been used regularly for more than ____
    a. 1 week
    b. 2 weeks
    c. 3 weeks
    d. 4 weeks

43. The drug approved for non-24-hour sleep–wake disorder is:
    a. Melatonin
    b. Tasimelteon
    c. Suvorexant
    d. Agomelatine

44. Zolpidem does not act on GABA-A receptor-containing:
    a. alpha 2 subunit
    b. alpha 3 subunit
    c. alpha 4 subunit
    d. alpha 5 subunit

45. The most common type of gamma subunit associated with benzodiazepine and Z drug effects is:
    a. gamma 1
    b. gamma 2
    c. gamma 3
    d. gamma 4

46. Which of the following matches is incorrect?
    a. Relapse = return of symptoms of an ongoing episode
    b. Rebound = increase of symptoms above the original baseline level
    c. Recurrence = entirely new episode
    d. None of the above

47. Which of the following is not a long-acting benzodiazepine?
    a. Chlordiazepoxide
    b. Clorazepate
    c. Flurazepam
    d. Bromazepam

48. Which of the following are the long-term consequences of chronic proton-pump inhibitor (PPI) use?

    i. Bone fractures; ii. dementia; iii. *Clostridium difficile*-associated diarrhea; iv. chronic kidney disease
    a. i., ii., and iii.
    b. i., iii., and iv.
    c. ii., iii., and iv.
    d. i., ii., iii., and iv.

49. Which of the following statements is not true?
    a. GABA-A receptors are five subunits of ligand-gated ion channels
    b. BDZs bind to a specific site present on GABA-A
    c. GABA-A receptors are not permeable to HCO_3^- ion
    d. GABA-A receptors are permeable to Cl^- ions

50. Which is incorrect about the relationship between memory impairment and benzodiazepine?
    a. Sensory and short-term memory are not affected by BZD
    b. BZDs impair episodic memory, but semantic memory is not impaired
    c. Impairments in implicit memory require relatively lower serum BZD levels than explicit memory impairments
    d. Flunitrazepam is used for drug-facilitated sexual assault (DFSA)

51. Which of the following is not true for prescription benzodiazepine dependence?
    a. Regular repeat prescriptions over a long period (months to years) pose a major risk of dependence
    b. Elderly females have a higher risk of dependence

c. Patients with physical and psychiatric problems and elderly residents of care homes are more vulnerable to prescription benzodiazepine dependence
d. Most patients who start on prescribed benzodiazepines rapidly escalate their dosage

52. All of the following statements about benzodiazepine withdrawal are true, *except*:
    a. BZD withdrawal is uncommon within 4 weeks of daily use
    b. BZD withdrawal occurs in about half of the patients treated daily for >4 months
    c. BZD withdrawal may last for 6–8 weeks
    d. Benzodiazepine withdrawal symptoms recover rapidly

53. Which of the following scales can be used for assessment of benzodiazepine withdrawal in pediatric patients?
    a. ASSIST
    b. CIWA-B
    c. Withdrawal Assessment Tool-1
    d. CIWA-Ar

54. Which of the following statements about benzodiazepine abuse is false?
    a. Most people who use nonprescription benzodiazepine use it with other drugs
    b. Opioid and benzodiazepine coadministration can lead to more severe respiratory depression
    c. Alcohol users do not usually develop tolerance to benzodiazepines
    d. Individuals receiving opioid agonist treatment commonly misuse benzodiazepines

55. All of the following are true about the relationship between BZD and sleep, *except*:
    a. BZDs increase the percentage of slow-wave sleep on chronic administration
    b. BZDs increase the REM latency
    c. BZD withdrawal increases the percentage of REM sleep
    d. Chronic administration of benzodiazepine enhances restful sleep

56. Which of the following statements about the National Survey on Extent and Pattern of Substance Use in India 2019 study is true?
    a. Around 10% of benzodiazepine users in India use the substance in a harmful or dependent pattern
    b. Mizoram has the highest prevalence of sedative use as well as dependence

c. A significant proportion of intravenous (IV) drug users use benzodiazepine as their choice of drug
d. Uttar Pradesh has the smallest number of people with problem use of sedatives

57. Carisoprodol:
i. a muscle relaxant; ii. is an opioidergic molecule; iii. structurally similar to meprobamate; iv. withdrawal profile which includes restlessness, aches and pain, insomnia, and anxiety.
a. All of the above are correct
b. Except ii. all are correct
c. Except iii. all are correct
d. Except iv. all are correct

58. Mr X is on opioid agonist treatment with buprenorphine–naloxone sublingual tablets (10 mg buprenorphine per day) for IV heroin use. He is irregular on his medication and uses heroin off and on. 2 days ago, he used heroin from a new dealer, and on chasing, his withdrawal symptoms did not improve. Subsequently, he consumed eight tablets of buprenorphine–naloxone (16 mg buprenorphine); as he had mild anxiety, he took 6-8 tablets of sleeping pills (clonazepam). Within 5 hours, he presented to the emergency with drowsiness, shallow breathing, and confusion; on examination, he had 87% oxygen saturation. What might be the cause of his clinical presentation?
a. Precipitate withdrawal due to buprenorphine
b. Inadvertent IV use of buprenorphine–naloxone combination
c. Respiratory depression due to concurrent use of opioids and benzodiazepine
d. Pulmonary granuloma as a complication of IV drug use

59. Regarding the management of high-dose benzodiazepine dependence, all are true, *except*:
a. One should gradually substitute the used benzodiazepine with a long-acting benzodiazepine like diazepam
b. The night dose will be substituted at the beginning, followed by the other dose
c. Benzodiazepine should be slowly tapered off over a couple of months
d. If there is insomnia, the night dose should be tapered off first, followed by the other doses

60. Compared to tramadol, tapentadol has:
a. Stronger opioid agonistic activity
b. Weaker serotonergic reuptake inhibition
c. Both of the above
d. None of the above

61. All of the statements about tapentadol are true, *except*:
    a. 50-mg tapentadol has equianalgesic action to 10-mg morphine
    b. Tapentadol has 50 times less affinity to μ-opioid receptors than morphine
    c. Tapentadol's norepinephrine reuptake inhibitor action has additional analgesic action
    d. History of monoamine oxidase inhibitor use within the previous 2 weeks is a contraindication of initiation of tapentadol

62. Regarding paradoxical reactions to benzodiazepines all are true, *except*:
    a. Characterized by increased talkativeness, emotional release, excitement, and excessive movement on administration of benzodiazepines
    b. Occur in <1% of patients
    c. Patients with psychiatric and/or personality disorders are at an increased risk
    d. Alcohol users are at a lower risk

63. All are true about the management of benzodiazepine intoxication, *except*:
    a. Respiratory depression is a common presentation warranting medical attention
    b. Symptomatic and supportive treatment is the mainstay
    c. Flumazenil is the drug of choice in comorbid poisoning with tricyclic antidepressant (TCA)
    d. Cardiac arrhythmia is a common side effect of flumazenil

64. According to the National Survey on Extent and Pattern of Substance Use in India 2019, all are true about pharmaceutical opioid use in India, *except*:
    a. In southern India, the prevalence of heroin use exceeds that of pharmaceutical opioid use
    b. Sikkim in northeast India has a higher prevalence of pharmaceutical opioid use than heroin use
    c. Pharmaceutical opioids are the second most commonly used opioid in India
    d. Prevalence of crude opium use is lower in India than heroin

65. All are designer benzodiazepines, *except*:
    a. Diclazepam
    b. Flubromazepam
    c. Pyrazolam
    d. Temazepam

66. Regarding the point-of-care (POC) detection test for benzodiazepine, all are true, *except*:
   a. POC test fails to detect oxazepam or its glucuronide conjugate
   b. Lorazepam, and flurazepam metabolism that does not result in oxazepam formation
   c. Estimated window of detection of diazepam and its metabolite in urine is up to 24 days
   d. Sertraline can cross-react with benzodiazepine during urine POC testing

67. Regarding barbiturate poisoning and its management, all are true, *except*:
   a. "Automatism phenomenon" is associated with fatal overdose
   b. Common signs are excessive CNS depression, confusion, coma, shallow and failing respirations, hypotension, cardiovascular collapse, renal shutdown, and bullous eruptions
   c. Routine gastric lavage has a limited role in management
   d. Forced alkaline diuresis should be started

68. The abuse potential of a prescription opioid is determined by all, *except*:
   a. Hydrophilicity
   b. Affinity to μ-receptor
   c. Route of administration
   d. Cost

69. All of the following are true for cyclobenzaprine, *except*:
   a. 5-HT2 receptor antagonist
   b. Most common signs of overdose are drowsiness and bradycardia
   c. Gastric lavage followed by activated charcoal is indicated in toxicity
   d. US FDA approved for muscle spasm.

70. Baclofen has been abused in all of the following routes, *except*:
   a. Oral
   b. Snorting
   c. Sublingual
   d. IV

71. Concomitant use of prescription opioid and skeletal muscle relaxants are associated with:
   a. Opioid overdose
   b. Muscle relaxant overdose
   c. Overdose of both
   d. Overdose of none

72. Which of the following has red- or orange-colored urine as a side effect?
   a. Cyclobenzaprine
   b. Chlorzoxazone
   c. Tizanidine
   d. Metaxalone

73. All of the following are true for loperamide abuse, *except*:
    a. Loperamide acts on the peripheral µ-receptor
    b. Cardiac toxicity is a major concern in overdose
    c. It is easily detected in drug screens
    d. Personal history of opioid use is common

74. The following is false for pentazocine:
    a. Introduced in the sixties in the last decade
    b. Marketed as a "nonnarcotic, nonaddictive" analgesic
    c. Its abuse is common among healthcare professionals
    d. High affinity only to the µ-receptor

75. Long-term abuse of PPIs leads to all, *except*:
    a. Increased gastric pH
    b. Hyperchlorhydria
    c. Congenital malformation
    d. Urinary tract infection

76. The most common substance use comorbidity with pregabalin misuse is:
    a. Alcohol
    b. Benzodiazepines
    c. Cannabis
    d. Opioid

77. The term "gabapentinoid" denotes:
    a. Gabapentin and pregabalin
    b. Gabapentin and pentazocine
    c. Gabapentin and retinoid
    d. Gabapentin and methylcobalamin

78. Pregabalin can be safely coprescribed with:
    a. Clozapine
    b. Sertraline
    c. Buprenorphine
    d. Clonazepam

79. All of the following are mechanisms of action of pregabalin, *except*:
    a. Binding to benzodiazepine binding sites at GABA-A receptors
    b. Binding to alpha 2-delta subunit of calcium channel
    c. Reducing the release of neurotransmitters
    d. None of the above

80. The most commonly abused anticholinergic is:
    a. Atropine
    b. Trihexyphenidyl
    c. Dicyclomine
    d. Scopolamine

81. According to the national survey on the extent and pattern of substance use in India, the prevalence of nonmedical, nonprescription use of sedatives–hypnotics is:
    a. 1–2%
    b. 2–3%
    c. 3–4%
    d. 14–15%

82. The following is true for melatonin:
    a. FDA-approved for jet lag disorder
    b. Production begins with phenylalanine
    c. Long-term use may cause poor semen quality
    d. Produced by the paraventricular nucleus of the hypothalamus

83. Concurrent abuse of opioids and benzodiazepines:
    a. Has strongest US-FDA warning
    b. Results increased emergency room visit
    c. Similar overdose potential to those who use only opioid
    d. All of the above

84. "Prescription metabolism" is:
    a. Drug interactions
    b. Polypharmacy
    c. Off-label prescription
    d. Deprescribing

85. "Polypharmacy" usually means the use of N or a greater number of drugs. The value of N is:
    a. 3
    b. 4
    c. 5
    d. 6

86. High-dose benzodiazepine dependence is characterized by all, *except*:
    a. Very high self-reported dose
    b. Severe withdrawal symptoms
    c. Frequent small dosing to maximize the effect
    d. Maintenance prescription of benzodiazepines in selected cases may reduce illicit benzodiazepine use

87. Which is true for the use of benzodiazepine in pregnancy?
    a. Benzodiazepines are freely permeable to the placental barrier and can potentially affect the fetus in the first trimester
    b. Low-dose chlorpromazine is the drug of choice for severe anxiety during pregnancy
    c. Both are true
    d. None of the above

88. All are true about benzodiazepine use in pregnancy and lactation, *except*:
    a. Diazepam may cause floppy baby syndrome during use in third trimester
    b. Diazepam is freely excreted in breast milk and may affect infants
    c. Lethargy, sedation, and weight loss are common features of benzodiazepine toxicity in children
    d. None of the above

89. Use of benzodiazepine in older adult:
    a. warrant caution, to be used with the lowest effective dose for the shortest possible time

b. Sedation, fall, and fracture are common complication of benzodiazepine use in the elderly
c. It may lead to hyperactivity and agitation
d. All are true

90. All are true for therapeutic dose benzodiazepine dependence, *except*:
    a. It occurs due to long-term prescription of benzodiazepines
    b. Commonly, benzodiazepine is prescribed for long periods to manage anxiety and depression
    c. Commonly, the users hike up the benzodiazepine dose
    d. Gradual dose reduction and minimal or brief intervention are the mainstay of treatment

91. All are true about the US opioid epidemic, *except*:
    a. It initiated an increase in the prescription of opioids for chronic pain
    b. Oxycodone was one of the major prescription opioids during the 90s
    c. The second and third waves of the opioid crisis were due to heroin overdose and stimulant-laced heroin use, respectively
    d. In 2017, the US declared opioid overdose as a public health emergency

92. Regarding monitoring prescription drug use, which one is true?
    a. Prescription database, if available, is not a reliable source
    b. Matching drug sales data with wastewater analysis gives an idea of the grey/black market of a prescription drug
    c. Drug diversion occurs exclusively from patients who sell their prescribed medication
    d. The most prevalent source of prescription drug misuse is the dark web

93. Regarding prescription drug misuse, all are true, *except*:
    a. The extent of misuse is proportional to the extent of clinical use and sale
    b. Patients legitimately using the drug are also at risk of misuse/abuse
    c. Prescription drugs with rapid onset of action and high potency are attractive for abuse or misuse
    d. The abuse potential of a drug is always readily observable when launching in the market

94. Which of the following has the shortest elimination half-life?
    a. Midazolam
    b. Temazepam
    c. Remimazolam
    d. Oxazepam

95. Which is not true about the cognitive side effects of benzodiazepine?
    a. Short-term memory loss in short-term use of benzodiazepine
    b. Anterograde amnesia
    c. Consolidation defect
    d. Long-term use of benzodiazepine is a risk factor for cognitive impairment in older adults

96. Which of the following is not true about the use of benzodiazepine in the first trimester?
    a. Increased rate of congenital anomaly is associated with benzodiazepine use
    b. Floppy baby syndrome is associated with BZD use in the first trimester
    c. Gastrointestinal (GI) malformation occurs in a higher-than-expected number of infants
    d. Orofacial aperture might be a congenital anomaly associated with BZD use

97. All are true about tele prescription of benzodiazepines, *except*:
    a. New prescriptions of clonazepam and clobazam are allowed with video consultation only as per Medical Council of India (MCI) recommendation in telemedicine practice guidelines 2020
    b. List A drugs require synchronous televideo consultation for prescription for the first time
    c. Any benzodiazepine can be prescribed during teleconsultation for alcohol withdrawal
    d. For a refill of clobazam in a case of epilepsy, only telephonic consultation is sufficient

98. Which of the following is considered a small quantity of diazepam under the Narcotic Drugs and Psychotropic Substances (NDPS) Act, 1985?
    a. 10 g and below
    b. 20 g and below
    c. 30 g and below
    d. 40 g and below

99. Which of the following is considered to be a commercial quantity of clonazepam under the NDPS Act, 1985?
    a. 50 g and above
    b. 100 g and above
    c. 150 g and above
    d. 200 g and above

100. Short-term benzodiazepine prescription is:
    a. <2 weeks
    b. <4 weeks
    c. <6 weeks
    d. <8 weeks

101. All are true about benzodiazepine prescription in generalized anxiety disorder (GAD), *except*:
    a. Benzodiazepine is a mainstay of treatment of mild-to-moderate GAD
    b. Benzodiazepine should be prescribed for not more than 2–4 weeks in GAD
    c. Pharmacotherapy is to be considered only after non-pharmacological management fails
    d. Patient needs to be informed about the addictive potential of benzodiazepine during prescribing

102. Regarding the deprescription of benzodiazepines, all are true, *except*:
    a. Deprescription aims to stop an already prescribed benzodiazepine through various approaches
    b. Slow taper with or without cognitive behavioral therapy (CBT) is a widely used deprescription approach
    c. Deprescription is associated with clinically significant sleep impairment during the initial 3 months
    d. Deprescription is associated with clinically significant sleep impairment during the initial 12 months

103. All are indications for benzodiazepine deprescription, *except*:
    a. Sleep difficulty in a patient with moderate depression under remission
    b. Patient with restless leg syndrome currently manageable with tablet Clonazepam
    c. 70-year-old male taking tablet clonazepam for sleep induction for the last 2 months
    d. A 50-year-old lady taking clonazepam for moderate GAD for 6 weeks

ANSWER KEY

1. c	2. d	3. b	4. b	5. d	6. c	7. b	8. c
9. b	10. a	11. b	12. b	13. d	14. c	15. a	16. d
17. d	18. c	19. a	20. c	21. d	22. b	23. a	24. d
25. a	26. c	27. d	28. c	29. c	30. a	31. a	32. d
33. b	34. a	35. c	36. a	37. c	38. c	39. d	40. c
41. d	42. b	43. b	44. d	45. b	46. d	47. d	48. d
49. c	50. c	51. d	52. d	53. c	54. c	55. a	56. a
57. b	58. c	59. d	60. c	61. a	62. d	63. c	64. a
65. d	66. a	67. c	68. a	69. b	70. d	71. a	72. b
73. c	74. d	75. b	76. d	77. a	78. b	79. a	80. b

81. b	82. c	83. c	84. d	85. c	86. c	87. c	88. d
89. d	90. c	91. c	92. a	93. d	94. c	95. a	96. b
97. c	98. b	99. b	100. b	101. a	102. d	103. b	

FURTHER READING

1. Ambekar A, Agrawal A, Rao R, Mishra AK, Khandelwal SK, Chadda RK on behalf of the group of investigators for the National Survey on Extent and Pattern of Substance Use in India. Magnitude of Substance Use in India. New Delhi: Ministry of Social Justice and Empowerment, Government of India; 2019
2. Bramness JG. Prescription drug abuse: Risks and prevention. In: El-Guebaly N, Carrà G, Galanter M (Eds). Textbook of Addiction Treatment: International Perspectives. 1st edition. New York: Springer; 2015. pp. 637-63.
3. Chakraborty K, Dan A. Clinical practice guidelines (CPG) for the management of sedative-hypnotic use disorders. In: Basu D, Dalal PK, (Eds). Clinical Practice Guidelines for the Assessment and Management of Substance Use Disorders, 1st edition. Hyderabad, Telangana: Indian Psychiatric Society; 2014. pp. 297-344.
4. Greenblatt HK, Greenblatt DJ. Designer Benzodiazepines: A Review of Published Data and Public Health Significance. Clin Pharmacol Drug Dev. 2019;8(3):266-9.
5. Mariani JJ. Sedative-, hypnotic-, or anxiolytic-related disorders. In: Sadock BJ, Sadock VA, Ruiz P (Eds). Kaplan and Sadock's Comprehensive Textbook of Psychiatry, 10th edition. Surrey, UK: Wolters Kluwer; 2017.
6. Mihic SJ, Mayfield J, Harris R. Hypnotics and sedatives. In: Brunton LL, Hilal-Dandan R, Knollmann BC (Eds). Goodman & Gilman's: The Pharmacological Basis of Therapeutics, 13 edition. New York: McGraw Hill; 2017.

CHAPTER 8

Gambling, Gaming, and Other Behavioral Addictions

Senjam Gojendra Singh, Mona Nongmeikapam,
Anuradha Moirangthem, Aworshim Muivah

1. "Compulsive gambling," later termed "pathological gambling," was first recognized in:
   a. DSM-5 (Diagnostic and Statistical Manual of Mental Disorders, Fifth Edition)
   b. DSM-III
   c. DSM-IV
   d. DSM-5 TR

2. Which is the first behavioral addiction to be recognized in DSM-5?
   a. Kleptomania
   b. Internet gaming disorder (IGD)
   c. Gambling disorder
   d. Pyromania

3. Pathological gambling was classified as an:
   a. Obsessive–compulsive related disorder
   b. Impulse control disorder
   c. Addiction disorder
   d. Other mental disorders

4. In DSM-5, gaming disorder comes under:
   a. Substance-related and addictive disorders
   b. Other conditions that may be a focus of clinical attention
   c. Unspecified other (or unknown) substance-related disorder
   d. Conditions for further study

5. IGD was figured for the first time in which diagnostic classification system?
   a. ICD-10 (International Classification of Diseases 10th Revision)
   b. DSM-5
   c. DSM-5 TR
   d. ICD-11

6. The first psychometric test to assess IGD was:
   a. Gaming Disorder Test
   b. Internet Gaming Disorder Test (IGD-20)
   c. Internet Gaming Disorder Scale—Short-Form (IGDS9-SF)
   d. Internet Gaming Disorder Scale (IGD-9)

7. Which was the first country to treat IGD clinically?
   a. South Korea
   b. China
   c. Canada
   d. Netherlands

8. IGD, as a formalized mental disorder, was included for the first time in:
   a. ICD-10
   b. ICD-11
   c. DSM-5
   d. DSM-5 TR

9. Gambling disorder is associated with all, *except*:
   a. Hypoactivation in the medial prefrontal cortex
   b. Hyperactivation in the ventral striatum
   c. Cortical grey thinning in the right prefrontal cortex
   d. Hypoactivation in the left dorsal anterior cingulate cortex

10. Impaired decision-making capacity in gambling disorder is attributed to:
    a. Hypoactivation in the ventral striatum
    b. Hypoactivation in the medial prefrontal cortex
    c. Hyperactivation in the ventral striatum
    d. Hyperactivation in the medial prefrontal cortex

11. For a diagnosis of gambling disorder, the individual should fulfill the diagnostic criteria in a:
    a. 12-month period
    b. 6-month period
    c. 10-month period
    d. 4-month period

12. According to the American Psychiatric Association, in the general population, the lifetime prevalence rate of gambling disorder is about
    a. 0.2–0.3%
    b. 0.4–1.0%
    c. 0.2–0.5%
    d. 0.6–0.9%

13. Specifiers for gambling disorder are all, *except*:
    a. In early/sustained remission
    b. Episodic/persistent
    c. Mild/ moderate/severe
    d. Early/late expression

14. Which of the following is not currently listed as a criterion for gambling disorder?
    a. Often gambles when feeling distressed
    b. Craving
    c. Tolerance
    d. Lies to conceal the extent of involvement with gambling

15. In gambling disorder, loss processing was associated with:
    a. Hypoactivation in the left dorsal anterior cingulate cortex
    b. Hyperactivation in the ventral striatum

c. Hyperactivation in the left dorsal anterior cingulate cortex
d. Hypoactivation in the ventral striatum

16. In gambling disorder, which neurotransmitter is involved in decision-making?
    a. Glutamatergic
    b. Dopaminergic
    c. Serotonergic
    d. Noradrenergic

17. _____ receptors are distributed widely in the mesolimbic system and are implicated in the hedonic aspects of reward processing in gambling disorder.
    a. Opioid
    b. Dopamine
    c. Noradrenaline
    d. Serotonin

18. As per the current evidence, which personality characteristic is implicated in gambling disorders?
    a. Transient impulse behavior
    b. Conscientiousness
    c. Impulsivity
    d. Openness to experience

19. Distorted cognitions in gambling disorder include all, *except*:
    a. Magnification of gambling skills
    b. Interpretative biases
    c. Temporal telescoping
    d. Catastrophizing

20. As per the etiological pathways model, all of the following individuals are involved/at risk, *except*?
    a. Behaviorally conditioned
    b. Extraverted impulsivist
    c. Emotionally vulnerable
    d. Antisocial impulsivist

21. The most widely studied non-pharmacological treatment modality for behavioral addictions is:
    a. Assertiveness skills training
    b. Dialectical behavioral therapy (DBT)
    c. Psychodynamic approaches
    d. Cognitive behavioral therapy (CBT)

22. One of the most well-known specialized inpatient and residential programs for internet addiction in the USA is:
    a. NO GAME
    b. Hope
    c. VirtDETOX
    d. reSTART

23. Behavioral and substance addictions have all of these similarities, *except*:
    a. Bimodal age distribution
    b. Onset in adolescence and young adulthood
    c. Chronic, relapsing patterns
    d. Craving

24. At present, the medications with the strongest empirical support in the treatment of gambling disorders are:
    a. Opioid receptor antagonists—naltrexone and nalmefene
    b. Selective serotonin reuptake inhibitors (SSRIs)—fluvoxamine and paroxetine
    c. Glutamatergic—N-acetyl cysteine
    d. Glutamate multimodal—acamprosate

25. Which scale has the largest research base for gaming disorder for its multiple positive features?
    a. YDQ (Young Diagnostic Questionnaire)
    b. IGUESS (Internet Game Use-Elicited Symptom Screen)
    c. GAS-7 (Game Addiction Scale-7 items)
    d. YIAT (Young Internet Addiction Test)

26. Which is a false statement?
    a. ICD-11 included gaming disorder into the substance and behavioral disorder chapter, and is inclusive of all game forms like online games, offline games, or other unspecified games
    b. ICD-11 and DSM-5 contain the diagnostic classification of hazardous use of games
    c. DSM-5 diagnostic criteria for gaming disorders are more detailed than the ICD-11, and therefore has good operability
    d. DSM-5, in addition, also comments on the prevalence, diagnosis, influencing factors, differential diagnosis, and comorbidity of online gaming disorder

27. Risk factors for gaming disorder are all, *except*?
    a. Social isolation   b. Younger age
    c. Depression   d. Alcohol use

28. Among internet-based games, _____ are the most complex and require the most intensive social interaction
    a. Single-player games
    b. Massively multiplayer online role-playing games (MMORPGs)
    c. First-person shooters (FPS)
    d. Strategy games

29. Domains of impulsivity, seen in gambling disorder, are all, *except*:
    a. Impulsive choice   b. Impulsive cognitive bias
    c. Reflection impulsivity   d. Impulsive reward

30. Increased metabolism in the middle orbitofrontal gyrus in gaming disorder may indicate:
    a. Compensatory cognitive processing
    b. Insensitivity to negative consequences

c. Higher reward sensitivity
d. Hyposensitivity to loss

31. Across behavioral addictions, all of the neural regions are consistently implicated, *except*:
    a. Ventral striatum
    b. Dorsal striatum
    c. Cingulate cortices
    d. Superior temporal lobe

32. _____ is associated with gaming disorder as both a risk factor and a comorbid condition.
    a. Depressive disorder
    b. Autism spectrum disorder
    c. Attention deficit hyperactivity disorder
    d. Obsessive–compulsive disorder

33. The "addictive" nature of gambling behavior and the disorder of pathological gambling can best be explained by theories of:
    a. Operant conditioning
    b. Classical conditioning
    c. Drive and neurotic impulses
    d. Self-psychology and pathological narcissism
    e. Habituation and sensitization

34. Many individuals with gambling disorders believe that:
    a. Money is the cause of their problems
    b. Money is the solution to their problems
    c. Money is the cause and the solution to their problems
    d. Money is the cause but not the solution to their problems

35. A pattern of "chasing one's losses" develops in which of the following disorder:
    a. Opioid use disorder
    b. Gambling disorder
    c. Internet addiction
    d. Cannabis use disorder

36. The period required to say that a person with a gambling disorder is in early remission is:
    a. 1–2 months
    b. 2–3 months
    c. 15 days to 1 month
    d. 3–12 months

37. Andrew, a 40-year-old, is suffering from a gambling disorder and was arrested by the police for criminal behavior to obtain money for gambling. In persons with gambling disorder like Andrew, criminal behavior is typically:
    a. Violent such as killing, assaulting people, etc.
    b. Nonviolent such as forgery, embezzlement, or fraud
    c. Both of the above
    d. Neither (a) nor (b)

38. All the following are true about compulsive shopping disorder, *except*:
    a. Lack of money could prevent compulsive shopping disorder from developing
    b. They often have comorbid psychiatric disorders, particularly mood, anxiety, substance use, and eating disorders
    c. Compulsive shoppers may more frequently have obsessive-compulsive, borderline, and avoidant personality types
    d. Not occurring only in the context of hypomanic or manic symptoms

39. A "whale" is a slang word used in relation to which of the following:
    a. Eating disorder
    b. Gaming disorder
    c. Both
    d. Gambling disorder

40. Previous editions of the DSM, before DSM-5, included pathologic gambling in:
    a. Substance use and addictive disorders
    b. Impulse control disorder
    c. Personality disorders
    d. None of the above

41. Amount of money spent wagering is _____ of gambling disorder.
    a. Indicative
    b. Not indicative
    c. Pathognomonic
    d. Both (a) and (b)

42. Certain areas of the brain gets activated in internet gaming. This occurs in the following brain regions, *except*:
    a. Frontal lobe–orbitofrontal area
    b. Nucleus accumbens
    c. Anterior cingulate area
    d. Ventromedial area

43. All of the following neurotransmitter systems, similar to substance use disorders, are implicated in the pathophysiology of behavioral addictions, *except*:
    a. Serotonin and dopamine
    b. Acetylcholine
    c. Noradrenaline
    d. Opioidergic

44. Taq1A1 allele of dopamine 2 receptor and Val158M are associated with substance use disorder. Its polymorphism has a higher incidence in which of the following:
    a. Gambling disorder
    b. Gaming disorder
    c. Compulsive shopping
    d. None of the above

45. For the following reasons, gaming disorder is categorized as an addiction-based mental illness:
    a. Gaming disorder is linked to the dopamine reward pathway and shares molecular mechanisms with drug use disorder

b. Those who suffer from gaming disorder may have a brain reaction to clues connected to games that is comparable to that of persons who suffer from drug use disorders
c. Medication and psychosocial therapies can help individuals with gaming disorders manage their symptoms while bolstering their physiology, cognition, and behavior
d. Pathological gambling and drug use disorders are linked to the genetic variants discovered in individuals with gaming problems
e. All of the above

46. The motivational enhancement therapy (MET)-CBT approach treatment for gaming disorder was used by Poddar and colleagues, which consisted of a series of stages that included the following steps:
    i. A contract stage with the patient, the parents, and the therapist (i.e., a behavior modification of gaming, reducing time spent online, and promoting healthy activities)
    i. A phase of reflection that includes the first sessions of rapport-building, a thorough interview, and case formulation
    ii. A preparatory phase, consisting of sessions presented in an understanding environment with an emphasis on psychoeducation, which includes controlling physiological and emotional arousal through relaxation techniques and analyzing the costs and benefits of gaming addiction

    The correct order of the above stages are:
    a. i., ii., iii.
    b. ii., iii., i.
    c. i., iii., ii.
    d. ii., i., iii.

47. Talismanic superstitions are cognitive distortions usually found in gambling disorders. It means:
    a. Exaggerating one's potential to win at gambling by thinking that owning particular items like a ring, makes one more likely to win
    b. Cognitive superstitions—the idea that winning odds can be influenced by specific mental states like prayer and positive predictions, etc.
    c. Both (a) and (b)
    d. None of the above

48. Attributional biases, which are a part of interpretative biases, found in gambling disorder means:
    a. The propensity to undervalue situational elements (such as chance or probability) and overstate dispositional factors (such as talents or aptitude) in order to explain victories
    b. The idea that following a run of defeats, a victory is finally due

c. The conviction that carrying on with gambling is the only way to make up for monetary losses
d. Assess gambling choices in retrospect as right or wrong depending on whether they result in wins or losses

49. Temporal telescoping, a distorted cognition present in problematic gamblers, is:
    a. Making gambling decisions based on interpretations or meanings assigned to subjectively salient or important cues
    b. Selectively recalling wins, especially large ones, and having difficulty recalling losses
    c. Belief that continuing to gamble is highly justifiable because losses are perceived as valuable learning experiences, which can ultimately lead to winning
    d. The belief that wins are nearer, temporally, than further, especially if the gambling relies on superstitious behavior or gambling systems to win

50. Several factors have been identified in the literature as being "motivations" for gambling. These include:
    a. Participating in gambling activities to demonstrate one's worth and get approval and social acceptance from others
    b. Relieve difficult and painful events/emotions (e.g., anger, depression, frustration, and anxiety)
    c. Win and be sociable
    d. All of the above

51. Hypersexuality or excessive sexual interest in males and females are respectively, known as:
    a. Nymphomania and satyriasis
    b. Satyriasis and nymphomania
    c. Paraphilia and pedophile
    d. Pedophile and paraphilia

52. All addictive disorders share common vulnerabilities from a neurobiological standpoint, which include:
    a. Impaired motivation–reward system
    b. Impaired affect regulation
    c. Impaired behavioral inhibition
    d. All of the above

53. The symptoms of sex addiction differ from sexual obsessions and compulsions primarily:
    a. In that the former is associated with sexual arousal and pleasure while the latter is typically accompanied not by sexual arousal but by anxiety

b. In that the former is associated not with sexual arousal but with anxiety, while the latter is typically accompanied by sexual arousal and pleasure
c. In that the former is associated with both arousal and anxiety while the latter is typically accompanied only by arousal
d. In that the former is associated only with arousal, not pleasure, while intrusive sexual thoughts typically accompany the latter

54. The key features that distinguish sex addiction from other patterns of sexual behavior are:
    a. The person is not able to control the sexual behavior
    b. The sexual behavior has significant harmful consequences and continues nonetheless
    c. Both (a) and (b)
    d. None of the above

55. Whether a pattern of sexual behavior qualifies as sex addiction is determined by:
    a. The type of behavior
    b. Its frequency
    c. Social acceptability
    d. How the behavior relates to and affects a person's life

56. Behavior mastery training is a set of techniques that persons suffering from sex addiction use on their own to help themselves refrain from enacting symptomatic behavior. It includes:
    a. Risk management
    b. Urge handling
    c. Symptom containment
    d. All of the above
    e. Only (b) and (c)

57. Risk management, which is a part of behavior mastery training for persons suffering from sex addiction, including:
    a. Teaching them to identify the factors that increase the likelihood of symptomatic behavior
    b. Training them to initiate protection against the influence of these factors
    c. Training them to initiate protection before the urges to engage in the behavior overwhelm their ability to recognize an effective defense
    d. All of the above

58. Paraphilic disorders include all of the following, *except*:
    a. Transvestism
    b. Voyeurism
    c. Exhibitionism
    d. Sexual masochism

59. The chronic obstacle to treatment success, now and in the future, for persons suffering from pathologic gambling are:
    a. The affected gambler's formidable resistance to getting help
    b. The affected gambler's formidable denial of the problem
    c. The affected gambler's alexithymic lack of introspection
    d. All of the above

60. Patients diagnosed with sex addiction are taught cognitive skills that they can employ to modify their thoughts. It includes:
    a. Accepting urges to engage in symptomatic sexual behavior as natural accompaniments to the healing process, not as signs of inadequacy
    b. Recognizing that urges are not imperatives to act but surface manifestations of effects
    c. Reviewing the benefits of refraining from symptomatic behavior and the potential negative consequences of engaging in that behavior
    d. All of the above

61. Which of the following are effective in managing compulsive shopping disorder?
    a. Group CBT, self-help books
    b. Financial counseling to help patients control compulsive spending
    c. Medicating for comorbid psychiatric disorders
    d. All of the above

62. The distinction between sex addiction and paraphilias include:
    a. Sex addiction can be diagnosed even when the criteria are unmet, while paraphilic disorders include conditions like transvestism
    b. There is no impaired ability to control the symptomatic behavior in sex addiction, whereas there is an impaired ability to control the symptoms in paraphilias
    c. Risk of harm to others due to symptomatic behavior is sufficient to warrant a diagnosis of paraphilic disorder but not sex addiction
    d. All of the above

63. All of the following are true, *except*:
    a. Gambling disorder (GD) is a psychiatric condition featuring recurrent, maladaptive gambling behavior
    b. GD causes clinically significant distress
    c. GD was reclassified into the "Substance-Related and Addictive Disorders" group of the DSM-5
    d. DSM-5 requires a minimum of 6 months to diagnose GD

64. DSM-5 criteria include at least 12 months of the following symptoms to diagnose gambling disorder, *except*:
    a. Need to gamble with an increasing amount of money to achieve the desired level of excitement
    b. Restlessness or irritability while attempting to cut down
    c. Preoccupation
    d. Part of a manic episode

65. Evidence-based treatment for gambling disorder includes all the following, *except*:
    a. Psychological Interventions like CBT are effective
    b. Individual or group therapy can reduce problem-gambling behavior, problem-gambling severity, and distress caused by problem-gambling
    c. Naltrexone can reduce gambling severity in problem gamblers
    d. All of the above

66. The following is true for dopamine agonists, *except*:
    a. May cause side effects such as impulse control disorders like binge eating, compulsive shopping, gambling disorder, or compulsive sexual behavior
    b. Are expressed predominantly in the brain limbic areas, which are implicated in addiction and impulse control disorders
    c. Treatment of restless leg syndrome with dopamine agonists leads to addiction and impulse control disorders
    d. Impulse control disorders in patients with restless leg syndrome are dose-dependent

67. All of the following are true, *except*:
    a. Abnormal reward-mediated processing is observed in Parkinson's disease
    b. Use of the dopamine 2/dopamine 3 selective receptor agonists is associated with an increased risk of diagnoses such as pathological gambling, compulsive buying, compulsive sexual behavior, and binge or compulsive eating
    c. Prevalence rates of behavioral addictions in dopamine agonist-treated patients with Parkinson's disease are much higher when compared to the general population
    d. Prevalence rates of behavioral addictions in dopamine agonist-treated patients with restless leg syndrome are negligible compared to the general population

68. All the following are proven effective in gambling disorder, *except*:
    a. CBT
    b. Exposure therapy with response prevention

c. Motivational interviewing and imaginal desensitization
d. DBT

69. According to DSM-5, the following are true, *except*:
   a. GD is a persistent and recurrent gambling pattern causing distress to the individual and impairment in their level of functioning
   b. GD is an impulse control disorder
   c. Patients with GD enjoy their gambling habit and experience distress on trying to cut down or stop their habit
   d. GD is only formally recognized behavioral addiction in the DSM-5 so far

70. The following are true about CBT in gambling disorder, *except*:
   a. CBT cannot be used with pharmacotherapy
   b. The cognitive component addresses the patients' thinking, attitudes, and belief systems which are considered the root of all behavioral problems
   c. The behavioral component aims to identify external triggers, practice their responses, and find and promote gambling alternatives
   d. Cognitive therapies aim to correct any cognitive abnormalities and challenge irrational thinking

71. All of the following are true, *except*:
   a. Exposure therapies with response prevention exposes the client to a gambling situation or gives them a clue and then teaches them to curb those desires in a more controlled acceptable manner
   b. Motivational intervention therapies counsels the client, challenges their uncertainties and works on enhancing their motivation to quit
   c. Psychodynamic psychotherapy works on resolving conflicts, reducing guilt or shame that may be associated with their current behavior
   d. Gamblers Anonymous is a core component of Alcoholics Anonymous

72. Which of the following is the first behavioral addiction as per the DSM-5?
   a. Gambling disorder
   b. Gaming disorder
   c. Porn addiction
   d. Compulsive shopping

73. Gambling disorder shares common features with those for substance use disorders. Which of the behavioral patterns is not true for both?
   a. Negatively reinforcing
   b. Lead to tolerance over time

c. Must meet two DSM-5 criteria to be considered a disorder
d. Related to clinically significant distress or impairment

74. Mr X has been a regular at the casino for more than a year. He also picked up drinking, much to the concern of his wife. He has been avoiding friends and family. However, Mr X claims that he only gambles for small fixed amounts and his work and financial commitments are not affected. What is the diagnosis?
    a. Social gambling
    b. Bipolar affective disorder, in mania
    c. Gambling disorder
    d. Pathological lying

75. Mrs A is a retired teacher. She has started visiting the local casino on a daily basis and most of the time, thinks and talks about gambling. She was even caught trying to steal casino chips on day. However, she keeps going back trying to recover the money previously lost. Mrs. A has features of:
    a. Social gambling
    b. Problematic gambling
    c. Gambling disorder
    d. Bipolar affective disorder, in mania

76. How would you define a social gambler?
    a. A person who needs to gamble more and more amounts of money to feel excited
    b. A person who gambles for fun on Holi or Diwali
    c. A person who believes gambling is a sort financial investment
    d. A person who steals money to gamble

77. What could lead to pathological gambling?
    a. Poor impulse control
    b. Use of alcohol
    c. Financial mismanagement
    d. All of the above

78. What are the steps that can be done as a psychiatrist to help a potential gambling addict:
    a. Set a limit on their spending
    b. Cut down their duration of gambling
    c. Mock their lack of self-control
    d. Medication their consent or knowledge

79. World Health Organization (WHO) recognizes which of the following activities as a mental disorder?
    a. Excess mobile use
    b. Oversleeping

c. Impaired control over gaming on mobile
d. Overeating

80. Ms. A says shopping is her primary social activity and entertainment. Though she works full-time, she shops three or more times a week. She buys clothing, shoes, makeup, jewelry, antiques, household electronics, and other items. She says that her shopping is spontaneous and impulsive. It gives her an emotional "rush". Occasionally, she feels guilty and returns or gives away purchased items. She is disappointed at her inability to control her shopping behavior and ashamed of the financial crises she has brought upon herself. What is she suffering from?
    a. Manic episode
    b. Hypomanic episode
    c. Compulsive shopping disorder
    d. Compulsive spending disorder

81. The following are true about IGD, *except*:
    a. Urbanization, lack of playgrounds, and technological developments contribute to the spread of internet-based games among adolescents
    b. These have increased depression, aggression, anxiety, violence, attention deficits, and impulsivity
    c. "IGD" is a disorder recognized by DSM-5
    d. Prevalence rates for IGD have been estimated to be <0.1% and 8.5% in adolescents and young adults

82. All the following are positive metacognitions in gaming disorder, *except*:
    a. "Gaming reduces worrying and will help me to control my thoughts"
    b. "Engaging with social media distracts my mind from problems"
    c. "Gaming relaxes me and helps me focus"
    d. "Once I start worrying, I cannot stop, so it is better to keep gaming"

83. Gaming Disorder, as per the WHO, is defined as all the following, *except*:
    a. A pattern of gaming behavior ("digital gaming or video gaming") characterized by impaired control over gaming
    b. Increasing priority given to gaming over other activities to the extent that gaming takes precedence over other interests and daily activities
    c. Continuation or escalation of gaming despite negative consequences
    d. A specifier under depressive disorders

84. Opposition toward the classification of "gaming disorder" as a mental health condition in the WHO's 11th revision of the International Classification of Diseases (ICD-11) is because of all the following reasons, *except*:
    a. The classification is intended to act as guidelines in many countries in determining healthcare policies, diagnosis, and treatment options. Hence, this "premature classification" could have a detrimental effect on treatment and policymaking
    b. Gaming addiction, as a disorder, could result in abuse of diagnosis and needs more study
    c. The addiction could also be a symptom of a deeper issue such as depression, and the new classification could result in merely treating the symptoms instead of the underlying issues
    d. The Indian online gaming industry was estimated to be worth $290 million as per a 2017 study and was projected to hit $1 billion by 2021

85. All these factors are common predictors for gaming motivation, *except*:
    a. Escapism—playing to avoid real-life difficulties
    b. Social interaction
    c. Thrill-seeking
    d. Unable to sleep

86. IGD is more with:
    a. Role-playing games (RPGs)
    b. Strategy (STR) games
    c. Action shooter (ACS) games
    d. Brain and skill (BRS) games

87. All the following are true about gaming disorder, *except*:
    a. Gaming takes precedence over other interests and daily activities
    b. There is continuation or escalation of gaming despite negative consequences
    c. For its diagnosis, behavior patterns need not result in significant impairment in personal, family, social, educational, occupational, or other important areas of functioning
    d. Symptoms have been evident for at least 12 months

88. All the following options suggest of gambling addiction, *except*:
    a. Continue to gamble even though they know it is problematic
    b. Gambling without realizing it is causing problems with the spouse or worsening sleep quality
    c. The addictive process becomes more valuable to a person.
    d. Gambling on annual family outings

89. Hypersexuality or sex addiction includes all of the below options, *except*:
    a. A persistent pattern of failure to control intense, repetitive sexual impulses or urges resulting in repetitive sexual behavior despite adverse consequences or deriving little or no satisfaction from it
    b. Obsessive behavior continues for 6 months or more
    c. Significant impairment or distress to functioning in other areas of life exists
    d. Watching porn

90. Sex addiction therapy involves all of the following, *except*:
    a. 12-step program Sex Addicts Anonymous
    b. CBT
    c. Psychotherapy
    d. Complete sex abstinence

91. All the following are true about porn addiction, *except*:
    a. Watching excessive amounts of porn, despite problems in relationships, work, or home life
    b. Continually lose track of time while watching porn
    c. Feelings of shame, guilt, or depression about porn viewing or trying to hide the fact that one watches it
    d. Recognized as a mental health diagnosis in the DSM-5

92. Which of the following is not an example of an intrinsically motivated activity?
    a. Eating and relishing their favorite snack
    b. Playing a game they enjoy
    c. Working hard to top an exam
    d. Reading their favorite novel

93. The two types of personalities according to Gray (1972) are:
    a. Individuals who get turned off by positive stimuli and get attracted to the reverse
    b. Individuals who like rewards and avoid aversion
    c. Individuals driven by personal gains and those who are altruistic
    d. Believers of the simple binary divisions of personality theory and nonbelievers

94. Motivation is not one of the following:
    a. Will or interest in a particular behavior
    b. Does not depend on emotion or cognition
    c. Preparatory period before any action
    d. Influenced by incentives

95. The revised reinforcement sensitivity theory by Gray and McNaughton, 2000 states that the behavioral inhibition system is to:
    a. Detect any goal conflict between reward and punishment
    b. Induce sensitivity to punishment
    c. Induce sensitivity to reward
    d. Induce inhibition of reward-seeking

96. Individuals with orbitofrontal cortex damage score low with the Iowa Gambling Task because:
    a. They make random choices
    b. They are inflexible with their thought process
    c. They are motivated by reward and not by losses
    d. They are very sensitive to punishment of loss

97. The incentive sensitization theory of addiction of Robinson and Berridge, 1993 states that a dopamine surge due to repeated drug use can cause:
    a. Hypersensitivity to the rewards of the drug usage
    b. Neural adaptations in the mesolimbic–dopamine pathway
    c. Hypersensitivity, for instance facial reactivity in laboratory rats secondary to pleasure
    d. Tolerance of drug rewarding mechanism

98. The DSM-IV-TR designates specific diagnostic criteria for behavioral addictions namely:
    a. Pathological gambling
    b. Kleptomania
    c. Internet addiction
    d. Compulsive shopping, pathologic skin-picking, sex addiction to name a few

99. Commonly exhibited behaviors in those with compulsive shopping disorders are:
    a. Irresistible urges, prompting spending by the patients
    b. They find shopping exciting, with transitory feelings of happiness and power
    c. Feelings of distress and guilt develop after shopping, need to hide purchases
    d. All of the above

100. Behavioral and substance addictions have many similarities, *except*
    a. Adolescence or young adulthood onset
    b. Incidence much higher than in older adults
    c. Chronic, recurrent behvioral pattern with multiple instances of quitting "spontaneously"
    d. Well-adjusted premorbid personality

101. Behavioral and substance addictions have phenomenological similarities, *except*:
    a. Excessive urge or craving before the onset of behavior
    b. Alleviation of anxiety and resultant elevation of mood
    c. Emotional dysregulation could aggravate craving
    d. Complicated withdrawal states from behavioral addictions

102. All of the following statements are true, *except*:
    a. Pathological gambling usually begins in childhood or adolescence
    b. Males tend to start earlier, mirroring the pattern of substance use disorders
    c. Higher rates of pathological gambling are observed in men, with a telescoping phenomenon observed in females (i.e., women have a later initial engagement in the addictive behavior but a foreshortened period from initial engagement to addiction)
    d. Gambling disorder is never comorbid with substance use disorders

103. Behavioral addiction and substance use disorder have the following commonalities:
    a. High impulsivity, sensation seeking behavioral pattern, and poor harm avoidance
    b. High levels of harm avoidance
    c. High harm avoidance and low impulsivity
    d. Worries about losing control over motor behaviors

104. Substance use disorders can commonly occur with:
    a. Pathological gambling
    b. Compulsive skin picking
    c. Compulsive shopping
    d. All of the above

105. Which of the following is true about compulsive shopping disorder?
    a. Onset is late adolescence to early adulthood
    b. Female-to-male ratio may be 9:1
    c. Shopping frequently, spending inappropriately, and fantasizing about future purchases
    d. All of the above

106. Patients with behavioral addictions and substance use disorders may have the following in common:
    a. They exhibit poor decision-making capacity
    b. They score low on inhibition tests
    c. They demonstrate cognitive flexibility
    d. They have excellent planning ability

107. The following neurobiological processes are involved in behavioral addiction:
    a. Multiple neurotransmitter systems such as serotonergic, dopaminergic, noradrenergic, and opioidergic
    b. Incoming reward pathway through the ventrotegmental area or the nucleus accumbens or the orbital frontal cortex (OFC) pathways
    c. The dopaminergic–mesolimbic pathway, originating from the ventrotegmental area up to the nucleus accumbens
    d. All of the above

108. The following have been found effective in the treatment of behavioral addiction:
    a. The 12-step self-administered method
    b. The motivational enhancement technique
    c. CBT
    d. All of the above

109. The following is/are approved in the treatment of behavioral addiction:
    a. Naltrexone
    b. SSRIs
    c. Behavioral therapy
    d. All of the above

ANSWER KEY

1. b	2. c	3. b	4. d	5. b	6. b	7. b	8. b
9. a	10. c	11. a	12. b	13. d	14. b	15. a	16. d
17. a	18. c	19. d	20. b	21. d	22. d	23. a	24. a
25. c	26. b	27. d	28. b	29. d	30. a	31. d	32. c
33. a	34. c	35. b	36. d	37. b	38. a	39. d	40. b
41. b	42. d	43. b	44. b	45. e	46. b	47. b	48. a
49. d	50. d	51. b	52. d	53. a	54. c	55. d	56. d
57. d	58. a	59. d	60. d	61. d	62. c	63. d	64. d
65. d	66. d	67. d	68. d	69. b	70. a	71. d	72. a
73. c	74. c	75. c	76. b	77. d	78. d	79. c	80. c
81. d	82. d	83. d	84. d	85. d	86. d	87. c	88. d
89. d	90. d	91. d	92. c	93. b	94. b	95. a	96. c
97. b	98. c	99. d	100. d	101. d	102. d	103. a	104. d
105. d	106. a	107. d	108. d	109. d			

FURTHER READING

1. American Psychiatric Association. Diagnostic and Statistical Manual of Mental Disorders, 3rd edition. Washington, DC: American Psychiatric Association; 1974.

2. American Psychiatric Association. Diagnostic and Statistical Manual of Mental Disorders, 5th edition. Washington, DC: American Psychiatric Association; 2013.
3. American Psychiatric Association. Diagnostic and Statistical Manual of Mental Disorders, fourth edition text revision (IV-TR). Washington, DC: American Psychiatric Association; 2000.
4. Aydın O, Güçlü M, Ünal-Aydın P, Spada MM. Metacognitions and emotion recognition in Internet Gaming Disorder among adolescents. Addict Behav Rep. 2020;12:100296.
5. Banyard P, Norman C, Dillon G, Winder B. (2023). Essential Psychology 3rd edition. [online] Available from https://study.sagepub.com/banyard3e [Last accessed December, 2023].
6. Bodor D, Ricijaš N, Filipčić I. Treatment of gambling disorder: review of evidence-based aspects for best practice. Curr Opin Psychiatry. 2021;34(5):508-13.
7. Boland R, Verduin M, Ruiz P. Kaplan & Sadock's Synopsis of Psychiatry, 12th edition. Philadelphia: Lippincott Williams & Wilkins; 2021.
8. Chamberlain SR, Lochner C, Stein DJ, Goudriaan AE, van Holst RJ, Zohar J, et al. Behavioural addiction—A rising tide? Eur Neuropsychopharmacol. 2016;26(5):841-55.
9. Gamaldo CE, Benbrook AR, Allen RP, Oguntimein O, Earley CJ. A further evaluation of the cognitive deficits associated with restless legs syndrome (RLS). Sleep Med. 2008;9(5):500-5.
10. Grant JE, Odlaug BL, Chamberlain SR. Neural and psychological underpinnings of gambling disorder: A review. Prog Neuropsychopharmacol Biol Psychiatry. 2016;65:188-93.
11. Grant JE, Potenza MN, Weinstein A, Gorelick DA. Introduction to Behavioral Addictions. Am J Drug Alcohol Abuse. 2010;36(5):233-41.
12. Grant JE. Impulse Control Disorders: A Clinician's Guide to Understanding and Treating Behavioral Addictions. New York: Norton Press; 2008.
13. Gupta D, Bennett-Li L, Velleman R, George S, Nadkarni A. Understanding internet gaming addiction in clinical practice. BJPsych Adv. 2021;27:383-93.
14. Han DH, Lee YS, Yang KC, Kim EY, Lyoo IK, Renshaw PF. Dopamine genes and reward dependence in adolescents with excessive Internet video game play. J Addict Med. 2007;1(3):133-8.
15. Ioannidis K, Hook R, Wickham K, Grant JE, Chamberlain SR. Impulsivity in Gambling Disorder and Problem Gambling: a meta-analysis. Neuropsychopharmacol. 2019;44(8):1354-61.
16. King DL, Chamberlain SR, Carragher N, Billieux J, Stein D, Mueller K, et al. Screening and assessment tools for gaming disorder: A comprehensive systematic review. Clin Psychol Rev. 2020;77:101831.
17. Lee S, Mysyk A. The medicalization of compulsive buying. Soc Sci Med. 2004;58(9):1709-18.
18. Leeman RF, Potenza MN. A targeted review of the neurobiology and genetics of behavioural addictions: an emerging area of research. Can J Psychiatry. 2013;58(5):260-73.
19. Liao Z, Chen X, Huang S, Huang Q, Lin S, Li Y, et al. Exploring the associated characteristics of Internet gaming disorder from the perspective of various game genres. Front Psychiatry. 2023;13:1103816.

20. Mestre-Bach G, Steward T, Granero R, Fernández-Aranda F, Mena-Moreno T, Vintró-Alcaraz C, Lozano-Madrid M, et al.Dimensions of Impulsivity in Gambling Disorder Sci Rep. 2020;10(1):397.
21. Nower L, Blaszczynski A, Anthony WL. Clarifying gambling subtypes: the revised pathways model of problem gambling. Addiction. 2022;117(7):2000-8.
22. Petry NM, Rehbein F, Ko CH, O'Brien CP. Internet Gaming Disorder in the DSM-5. Curr Psychiatry Rep. 2015;17(9):72.
23. Poddar S, Sayeed N, Mitra S. Internet gaming disorder: Application of motivation enhancement therapy principles in treatment. Indian J Psychiatry. 2015;57(1):100-1.
24. Raimo S, Cropano M, Trojano L, Santangelo G. The neural basis of gambling disorder: An activation likelihood estimation meta-analysis. Neurosci Biobehav Rev. 2021;120:279-302.
25. Raylu N, Oei TP. A Cognitive Behavioural Therapy Programme for Problem Gambling. Therapist Manual, 1st edition. New York: Routledge; 2010. p. 10.
26. Ribeiro EO, Afonso NH, Morgado P. Non-pharmacological treatment of gambling disorder: a systematic review of randomized controlled trials. BMC Psychiatry. 2021;21(1):105.
27. Sadock BJ, Sadock VA, Ruiz P. Kaplan & Sadock's Comprehensive Textbook of Psychiatry, 10th edition. Philadelphia: Lippincott Williams & Wilkins; 2017.
28. Saunders JB, Hao W, Long J, King DL, Mann K, Fauth-Bühler M, et al. Gaming disorder: Its delineation as an important condition for diagnosis, management, and prevention. J Behav Addict. 2017;6(3):271-9.
29. Toneatto T, Ladoceur R. Treatment of pathological gambling: a critical review of the literature. Psycol Addict Behav. 2003;17:284-92.
30. Wang Q, Ren H, Long J, Liu Y, Liu T. Research progress and debates on gaming disorder. Gen Psychiatr. 2019;32(3):e100071.
31. Weintraub D, Koester J, Potenza MN, Siderowf AD, Stacy M, Voon V, et al. Impulse control disorders in Parkinson disease: a cross-sectional study of 3090 patients. Arch Neurol. 2010;67(5):589-95.
32. World Health Organization. (2021). International Statistical Classification of Diseases and Related Health Problems. International Classification of Diseases 11th Revision. [online] Available from https://www.who.int/standards/classifications/classification-of-diseases [Last accessed December, 2023].
33. Yau YH, Potenza MN. Gambling disorder and other behavioral addictions: recognition and treatment. Harv Rev Psychiatry. 2015;23(2):134-46.

CHAPTER 9

Miscellaneous

Gayatri Bhatia, Ankita Chattopadhyay, Rahul Mathur

ANABOLIC ANDROGENIC STEROIDS

1. Normal testosterone plasma concentrations for *men* range from:
   a. <100 ng/mL
   b. 300–1,000 ng/dL
   c. 1,000–2,000 ng/mL
   d. >2,000 ng/mL

2. All of the following effects can be seen due to anabolic steroids, *except*:
   a. Testicular atrophy
   b. Sterility
   c. Hyperprolactinemia
   d. Gynecomastia

3. The prevalence of hypomania or a mania among anabolic steroid misusers is:
   a. 1%
   b. 10%
   c. 20%
   d. 30%

4. False statement regarding nandrolone decanoate is:
   a. High rates of liver toxicity
   b. High anabolic to androgenic effect ratio
   c. It is a progestin
   d. Suppresses hypothalamic–pituitary–testicular axis

5. Which was the first anabolic androgenic steroid synthesized?
   a. 19-nortestosterone
   b. Methyltestosterone
   c. Trenbolone hexahydrobenzylcarbonate
   d. Boldenone undecylenate

6. All of the following are Food and Drug Administration (FDA)-approved indications for use of anabolic steroids, *except*:
   a. Primary hypogonadism
   b. Cryptorchidism
   c. Growth failure
   d. Vanishing testis syndrome

7. Anabolic androgenic steroids are included in which schedule of the Drug Enforcement Administration?
   a. Schedule I
   b. Schedule II
   c. Schedule III
   d. Schedule IV

8. All of the following are oral preparations of anabolic androgenic steroids, *except*:
   a. Oxymetholone
   b. Oxandrolone
   c. Testosterone enanthate
   d. Methandrostenolone

9. Which of the following is correctly defined?
    a. "Cycling" is using more than one steroid at a time to maximize lean muscle mass, weight gain, and strength increases
    b. "Stacking"—the user follows a cycle of building up to a peak dose and then tapering back down toward the end of the cycle, hoping to allow the body's hormonal system time to recuperate and maintain homeostasis
    c. "Pyramiding"—the user takes the steroid for 4–12 weeks and then stops for a variable period, after which use is resumed
    d. None of the above

10. Among the following personality profiles, which is *least* likely to abuse anabolic steroids?
    a. Anankastic
    b. Histrionic
    c. Borderline
    d. Antisocial

ARECA NUT

11. Areca nut is used in all, *except*:
    a. Khaini
    b. Gutka
    c. Pan masala
    d. Betel quid

12. The following alkaloids are found in Areca nut, *except*:
    a. Arecoline
    b. Cotinine
    c. Arecaidine
    d. Guvacine

13. Which of the following is *not* true?
    a. Betel quid itself, with or without tobacco, is a group I carcinogen
    b. Areca nut used in any form causes only oral cancer
    c. Areca nut can cause potentially malignant oral disorders such as leukoplakia and erythroplakia
    d. Chewing areca nut is an important etiological factor for developing oral submucosal fibrosis

14. Which of the following is *not* true?
    a. Educational interventions focused on preventing areca nut use have been found effective
    b. Lack of awareness about areca nut harms is one of the main barriers to treatment-seeking
    c. Pharmacological interventions are established for areca nut use disorder
    d. Psychological interventions are being tried for areca nut use disorder, using techniques like cognitive behavior intervention and culturally tailored behavior change interventions

15. All of the following are true, *except*:
    a. Arecoline stimulates various brain receptors, promoting physical dependence
    b. Areca nut can cause or worsen conditions such as myocardial infarction and cardiac arrhythmias
    c. Areca nut is helpful for patients with type 2 diabetes and prevents metabolic syndrome
    d. Areca nut use (areca with or without tobacco) remains an orphan addiction

CAFFEINE

16. Which of the following is *not* true about caffeine metabolism?
    a. Metabolism occurs in the liver through the cytochrome P450 pathway, especially the cytochrome CYP1A2
    b. Disulfiram has been shown to impair caffeine metabolism
    c. During pregnancy, the half-life of caffeine increases
    d. Smokers seem to metabolize caffeine slowly

17. All of the following are metabolites of caffeine, *except*:
    a. Theobromine
    b. Thebaine
    c. Theophylline
    d. Paraxanthine

18. Which of the following is not true in diagnoses related to caffeine in the DSM-5 (Diagnostic and Statistical Manual of Mental Disorders, Fifth Edition)?
    a. Caffeine intoxication
    b. Caffeine withdrawal
    c. Other caffeine-induced disorders
    d. Caffeine use disorder is included in substance-related and addictive disorders

19. Diagnosis of caffeine withdrawal in ICD-10 (International Classification of Diseases 10th Revision) includes all, *except*:
    a. Lethargy and fatigue
    b. Insomnia or hypersomnia
    c. Psychomotor retardation or agitation
    d. Decreased appetite

20. Other caffeine-induced disorders in DSM 5 include:
    a. Caffeine-induced anxiety disorders
    b. Caffeine-induced sleep disorders
    c. Both
    d. None

21. Which of the following concerning caffeine in ICD 11 is not true?
    a. Single episode of harmful use of caffeine
    b. Harmful pattern of use of caffeine
    c. Caffeine withdrawal
    d. Caffeine is included under stimulants

22. Which of the following is *not* true?
    a. Regular consumption of coffee has been found to decrease the incidence of type 2 diabetes
    b. Caffeine influences the metabolism of uric acid and the occurrence of gout
    c. Caffeine is considered a doping substance controlled by the World Anti-Doping Agency (WADA)
    d. Coffee has been shown to protect against Parkinson's disease

23. All of the following are true about the management of caffeine intoxication, *except*:
    a. Cardiovascular or neurologic toxicities are common
    b. Sinus tachycardia occurs but does not require any intervention
    c. Dialysis or hemofiltration may be necessary for extremely high caffeine levels
    d. Gastric lavage should always be considered

24. Proposed criteria for caffeine use disorder in DSM-5 include a problematic pattern of use of caffeine manifested by at least three of the following criteria, *except*:
    a. Withdrawal
    b. Continued use despite knowledge of harm due to caffeine
    c. Tolerance
    d. Persistent desire to cut down on caffeine use

25. Which of the following statements about caffeine withdrawal is false?
    a. The main problems are fatigue, lack of concentration, or headache
    b. Caffeine withdrawal is mostly self-limited
    c. General interventions such as rest, physical activity, and fluid and electrolytes are recommended
    d. Analgesics are contraindicated

NEW PSYCHOACTIVE SUBSTANCES

26. What is *false* about new psychoactive substances (NPSs)?
    a. These mimic the pharmacological effects of established illicit drugs
    b. These are chemically similar to established illicit drugs
    c. These are difficult to detect in body fluids
    d. These are safer for consumption than illicit drugs

27. What is *true* regarding NPSs?
    a. These are synthetic compounds with psychoactive effects similar to controlled substances
    b. They have lower abuse potential compared to their parent compound
    c. The United Nations drug conventions do not control these
    d. These are commonly used in developing countries as they are cheaper
28. Which group of drugs mimic the effect of amphetamines?
    a. Synthetic cathinone
    b. Phenethylamines
    c. Synthetic cannabinoids
    d. Tryptamines
29. Psychedelics are all, *except*:
    a. Hallucinogens
    b. $5HT_{2A}$ agonists
    c. N-methyl-D-aspartate (NMDA) agonists
    d. Entactogens
30. Which of the following are *not* psychedelics?
    a. Psilocybin
    b. Lysergic acid diethylamide
    c. 1-benzylpiperazine (BZP)
    d. Diemethyltryptamine
31. The mechanism of action of ketamine as an antidepressant is:
    a. GluN2B-selective NMDA receptor (NMDAR) inhibition
    b. Inhibition of NMDA-dependent burst activity of lateral habenular neurons
    c. Preferential inhibition of the NMDAR on GABAergic interneurons
    d. All of the above
32. The most popular group of NPSs used in India is:
    a. Amphetamine-type stimulants
    b. Synthetic opioids
    c. Synthetic cannabinoids
    d. Hallucinogens
33. Marketing advantages of synthetic over plant-based NPSs are all, *except*:
    a. Quicker production time
    b. Pharmacological effects and interactions are largely understood
    c. It can be manufactured close to end markets
    d. All of the above
34. "Bad trip" is characterized by:
    a. Anxiety and panic-like symptoms
    b. Disorganized thinking
    c. Intense depression
    d. Delirium

35. FDA-approved psychedelic for the treatment of post-traumatic stress disorder (PTSD) is:
    a. Ketamine
    b. Psilocybin
    c. MDMA (methylenedioxymethamphetamine)
    d. DMT (N,N-dimethyltryptamine)

36. The global prevalence of use of MDMA as of 2021–2022 is:
    a. 0.4%   b. 1%
    c. 2%   d. 2.5%

37. FDA approval was given to esketamine in 2019 for the treatment of:
    a. Treatment-resistant schizophrenia
    b. Treatment-resistant depression (TRD)
    c. Intractable epilepsy
    d. Severe depression without psychotic features

DRUG USE IN SPECIAL POPULATIONS

38. What is the prevalence (%) of current alcohol use in those between 10 and 17 years in India?
    a. 0.5   b. 1.3
    c. 1.6   d. 2.5

39. T-ACE (Tolerance, Annoyed, Cut down, and Eye-opener) screening instrument is commonly used for screening for risk drinking in which population group?
    a. Obstetrics and gynecology   b. Adolescents
    c. Prisoners   d. Elderly

40. Which of the following is *not* a feature of fetal alcohol syndrome?
    a. Micrognathia   b. Thin upper lip
    c. Flattened face   d. Macrocephaly

41. The prevalence (%) of inhalant use disorders in adolescents in India is?
    a. 0.07   b. 1.2
    c. 1.5   d. 2.0

42. Pharmacological treatment of choice for childhood nicotine dependence:
    a. Nicotine replacement therapy
    b. Varenicline
    c. Bupropion
    d. Nortriptyline

Miscellaneous

UNITED NATIONS DRUG CONVENTIONS

43. Which of the following countries is *not* a part of the Golden Triangle?
    a. Myanmar
    b. Laos
    c. Thailand
    d. Cambodia

44. The secretariat of the International Narcotics Control Board (INCB) is located at:
    a. Vienna
    b. Geneva
    c. Paris
    d. Bangkok

45. Which of the following is *incorrect* regarding the first International Opium Convention?
    a. It took place in 1912
    b. It was held in Hague, Netherlands
    c. To curb the excesses of an unregulated system of free trade
    d. It laid down an enforceable multilateral treaty

46. The number of articles in the Single Convention on Narcotic Drugs, 1961 is:
    a. 31
    b. 41
    c. 51
    d. 61

47. Which of the following options is *false* regarding Convention on Psychotropic Substances 1971?
    a. It has 33 articles
    b. It was adopted in Geneva, Switzerland, in 1971
    c. Schedule I is the most restrictive
    d. It has 184 signatories

48. Which of the following options is *false* regarding the INCB?
    a. It has 23 members
    b. It was established in 1968 in accordance with the Single Convention on Narcotic Drugs, 1961
    c. India is a signatory to treaties laid down by INCB
    d. It is a quasi-judicial body

49. Which of the following pairs are *wrongly* matched?
    a. Schedule I—LSD
    b. Schedule II—MDMA
    c. Schedule III—Buprenorphine
    d. Schedule IV—Phenobarbital

50. The World Drug Report is an annual publication that analyzes market trends, compiling detailed statistics on drug markets. Which agency is tasked with publishing the World Drug Report?
    a. International Narcotics Control Bureau
    b. Expert Committee on Drug Dependence

c. Economic and Social Council
d. United Nations Office on Drugs and Crime (UNODC)

51. The World Food Programme and the UNODC work in *collaboration* to achieve which of the following?
    a. Prevention of substance use among adolescents
    b. Eradicating hunger in vulnerable populations
    c. HIV prevention and control, decriminalization, and zero discrimination against people who use drugs
    d. Financial assistance in research activities and implementation of drug laws in member states

52. Which drugs were *added* to Schedule IV of the Convention on Psychotropic Substances of 1971 in 2020?
    a. Mirtazapine   b. Etizolam
    c. Baclofen   d. Trazodone

HISTORICAL ASPECTS OF SUBSTANCE USE

53. Opium is known to originate from which country?
    a. China   b. Egypt
    c. Turkey   d. India

54. When was the opium trade banned in China?
    a. 1553   b. 1799
    c. 1837   d. 1845

55. Where was tobacco first cultivated?
    a. Africa   b. Australia
    c. North America   d. Southeast Asia

56. All species of cannabis produce tetrahydrocannabinol, *except*:
    a. *Cannabis sativa*   b. *Cannabis brasiliensis*
    c. *Cannabis ruderalis* d. *Cannabis indica*

57. Which is *not* a dry state?
    a. Gujarat   b. Maharashtra
    c. Bihar   d. Nagaland

58. The legal driving limit for alcohol in India is:
    a. 30 mg/100 mL of blood   b. 50 mg/100 mL of blood
    c. 75 mg/100 mL of blood   d. 80 mg/100 mL of blood

59. Recreational cannabis is legal in all these countries, *except*:
    a. Canada   b. Madagascar
    c. Thailand   d. Uruguay

60. The sale of e-cigarettes is *banned* in:
    a. Sri Lanka   b. Pakistan
    c. Bangladesh   d. India

61. Which of the following festivals is associated with bhang?
    a. Diwali
    b. Bihu
    c. Holi
    d. Onam

62. In traditional medicine, opium was used for the treatment of all, *except*:
    a. Diarrhea
    b. Unexplained fever
    c. Poor appetite
    d. Aches and pains

NARCOTIC DRUGS AND PSYCHOTROPIC SUBSTANCES ACT

63. The Narcotic Drugs and Psychotropic Substances (NDPS) Act is administered by the:
    a. Ministry of Health and Family Welfare (MOHFW)
    b. Ministry of Social Justice and Empowerment (MOSJE)
    c. Ministry of Finance
    d. Ministry of Home Affairs

64. NDPS Act came into effect from:
    a. 1985
    b. 1988
    c. 1989
    d. 1995

65. India's approach toward narcotic drugs and psychotropic substances is based on which article of the Constitution of India?
    a. Article 44
    b. Article 47
    c. Article 42
    d. Article 43

66. Narcotic drugs, according to the NDPS Act, include all, *except*:
    a. Coca leaf
    b. Opium
    c. Poppy straw
    d. Poppy seeds

67. Which of the following is *not* an essential narcotic drug (END)?
    a. Methadone
    b. Buprenorphine
    c. Morphine
    d. Fentanyl

68. Immunity from prosecution to addicts volunteering for treatment is included in which section of the NDPS Act?
    a. Section 47
    b. Section 47a
    c. Section 27
    d. Section 64a

69. NDPS Act amendments occurred in all of the following years, *except?*
    a. 1989
    b. 2001
    c. 2004
    d. 2014

70. All of the following are psychotropics in the NDPS Act, *except*:
    a. Diazepam
    b. Tramadol
    c. Methadone
    d. Buprenorphine

Miscellaneous

71. Which of the following is *not* included in the NDPS Act?
    a. Bhang
    b. Charas
    c. Hashish
    d. Ganja
72. NDPS Act applies to:
    a. Citizens of the whole of India
    b. All citizens of India outside India
    c. All persons on ships and aircraft registered in India
    d. All of the above
73. A person was caught possessing 1 kg of Ganja. What will be the punishment according to the NDPS Act?
    a. Rigorous imprisonment of up to 1 year
    b. Fine up to Rs 10,000
    c. Can be both
    d. No punishment for first-time offenders
74. Section 39 of the NDPS Act refers to:
    a. Power of court to release certain offenders on probation
    b. It concerns offences related to a small quantity of any narcotic drug or psychotropic substance
    c. The court can direct the offender to be released to undergo medical treatment
    d. All of the above
75. Responsibilities of an Officer in Charge (OIC) of a Recognized Medical Institution (RMI) about ENDs include:
    a. Dispensing ENDs to patients registered with the RMI
    b. Maintenance of stock of ENDs for 3 months in the RMI
    c. Record keeping for 2 years for each patient
    d. All of the above
76. The Central Bureau of Narcotics issues licenses for legal opium cultivation in all these states, *except*:
    a. Uttar Pradesh
    b. Madhya Pradesh
    c. Rajasthan
    d. Haryana
77. According to NDPS policy, which of the following is *true* in prison?
    a. All injection drug users (IDUs) must be compulsorily de-addicted
    b. They should be given opioid substitution therapy
    c. They can be provided with fresh needles and syringes
    d. None of the above

DRUG DE-ADDICTION PROGRAMME OF INDIA

78. The "Drug De-Addiction Programme" (DDAP) was initiated in?
    a. 1988
    b. 1996
    c. 2004
    d. 2014

79. The nodal ministry for demand reduction is:
    a. Ministry of Health and Family Welfare
    b. Ministry of Social Justice and Empowerment
    c. Department of Revenue
    d. Ministry of Labor

80. The national nodal center for DDAP is?
    a. NDDTC, AIIMS New Delhi
    b. PGIMER, Chandigarh
    c. CIP, Ranchi
    d. RIMS, Imphal

81. Nasha Mukt Bharat Abhiyan under the DDAP is implemented by?
    a. Ministry of Health and Family Welfare
    b. Ministry of Social Justice and Empowerment
    c. Ministry of Home Affairs
    d. Ministry of Human Resource Development

82. Which of the following is *not* an objective of the DDAP?
    a. Provide affordable treatment for substance use disorders
    b. Making treatment easily accessible
    c. Training of primary care physicians to treat substance use disorders
    d. Providing evidence-based treatment

NATIONAL AIDS CONTROL PROGRAMME

83. The relative risk of contracting HIV among people who inject drugs (PWID) as compared to the general population is:
    a. Five times
    b. Ten times
    c. Twenty times
    d. Thirty times

84. The highest number of PWID are recorded from which state in India?
    a. Punjab
    b. Uttar Pradesh
    c. Haryana
    d. Mizoram

85. As per the Integrated Biological and Behavioral Surveillance, 2014–15, the prevalence of HIV among PWID in India is:
    a. 5%
    b. 10%
    c. 15%
    d. 20%

86. As per the National AIDS Control Programme, which is *not* a recognized high-risk group (HRG) for HIV infection?
    a. Long-distance truckers
    b. Female sex workers
    c. PWID
    d. Children of people living with HIV

87. The risk of transmission of HIV with needle sharing is:
    a. >1 per 100,000 exposures
    b. 10 per 100,000 exposures
    c. 20 per 100,000 exposures
    d. 40 per 100,000 exposures
88. All of the following are targeted interventions for HIV prevention among PWID, *except*:
    a. Needle syringe exchange
    b. Opioid substitution
    c. Antiretroviral treatment
    d. Rehabilitation and community reintegration
89. Needle syringe exchange in India works on the principle of:
    a. One-for-one exchange
    b. Point of sales system
    c. Less than 100% exchange
    d. Distribution without exchange
90. The main agent for opioid substitution therapy in India is:
    a. Methadone
    b. Buprenorphine
    c. Tramadol
    d. Morphine
91. Current targets envisaged for achievement under the "National Strategic Plan for HIV, AIDS and STI, 2017–2024" are:
    a. 95-95-95: 95% of the population tested for HIV, 95% of those found positive on antiretroviral therapy, and 95% of those showing viral load suppression
    b. 90% coverage of condom distribution program
    c. 60% reduction in new HIV infections
    d. 75% reduction in new HIV mortality
92. Key populations for HIV include all, *except*:
    a. Hijra/transgender
    b. Migrant population
    c. Men who have sex with men
    d. Family members of PWID

DRUG-RELATED LAWS AND POLICIES—INTERNATIONAL SCENARIO

93. "War on Drugs" was coined by:
    a. Roosevelt
    b. Nixon
    c. Obama
    d. Reagan
94. MORE Act, 2022 stands for:
    a. Morphine and Other Opioid Rehabilitation and Experimentation Act
    b. Methadone Opportunity Rehabilitation and Expungement Act
    c. Marijuana Opportunity Reinvestment and Expungement Act
    d. Marijuana Opportunity Rehabilitation and Expungement Act

95. The Iron Law of Prohibition states that:
    a. As law enforcement becomes more intense, the potency of prohibited substances increases
    b. If drugs are legalized, consumers will wean off higher-potency forms
    c. If a drug's cost is raised, fewer people will initiate its regular use
    d. The youth population tends to shift from easily available drugs to prohibited drugs as they age

96. All are true about harm reduction, *except*:
    a. The aim is to prevent adverse consequences of drug use
    b. Harm reduction focuses on the responsible continuation of drug use
    c. Harm reduction practices are meant for clients not ready to quit drug use
    d. Harm reduction practices normalize drug use in society

97. All of the following harm reduction practices are followed in Southeast Asia region, *except*:
    a. Needle syringe exchange
    b. Opioid substitution
    c. Safe injection sites
    d. Take-home naloxone distribution

CASE-BASED SCENARIOS

98. David consumed 90 mL of whiskey at a house party within 1 hour. After how many hours will he be considered *safe* to drive?
    a. 1 hour
    b. 3 hours
    c. 6 hours
    d. 12 hours

99. A person was presented in high court under charges of forcefully injecting a minor girl with heroin with the intent of sexually abusing her. He was apprehended before he could proceed with sexual activity. Under what act will he be convicted?
    a. Narcotic Drugs and Psychotropic Act
    b. Protection of Children against Sexual Offenses Act
    c. Juvenile Justice Act
    d. The HIV and AIDS (Prevention and Control) Act

100. A young college student was brought to the Emergency Medicine Department by his batchmates after being seen to behave abnormally for the last 1 hour. He was highly agitated and fearful, pointing toward the exit where he saw an army of black-clad men coming to kill him. There was no history indicative of an ongoing psychiatric illness.

He had an unstable gait, profuse sweating, tachycardia, and dilated pupils. What will be the immediate line of management?
a. Stabilize vitals, reassure, send urine for toxicology screening, and maintain a calm environment free of unnecessary stimulation
b. Sedate the patient using benzodiazepines, wait for him to wake up and take a detailed history
c. Start antipsychotics to manage the agitation and fearfulness
d. None of the above

ANSWER KEY

Anabolic Androgenic Steroids

1. a. 300–1,000 ng/dL—the normal testosterone range for men is typically between 300–1,000 ng/dL. Normal testosterone range for women is 15–70 ng/dL of blood.
2. c. Hyperprolactinemia—all of the listed effects can be seen due to anabolic steroids except hyperprolactinemia.
3. b. 10%—the prevalence of hypomania or mania among anabolic steroid misusers is approximately 10%.
4. a. Hepatotoxicity risk with nandrolone decanoate is quite low.
5. a. 19-nortestosterone was the first anabolic androgenic steroid synthesized in 1953.
6. c. Growth failure—All of the listed options are FDA-approved indications for the use of anabolic steroids except growth failure.
7. c. Schedule III—Anabolic Androgenic Steroids are included in Schedule III of the DEA. Reference:
8. c. Testosterone enanthate—All of the options are oral preparations of anabolic androgenic steroids except testosterone enanthate, which is an intramuscular (IM) injectable preparation.
9. d. None of the above. "Cycling" is the process of rotating between "on" and "off" periods of steroid intake. "Stacking" is the process of using more than one steroid (oral with injectable or more androgenic with more anabolic) agents at a time. "Pyramiding" is starting with a small dose of a steroid and gradually increasing that over time (until the user reaches a peak at mid-cycle) before tapering off (gradually reducing the dosage or frequency down to zero) to complete a cycle.
10. a. Anankastic personality

Areca Nut

11. a. Khaini. People use areca nut alone or in a betel quid comprising ingredients such as betel leaf, slaked lime, and tobacco. Areca nut is used in commercial products such as gutka and pan masala.
12. b. Cotinine. Arecoline, arecaidine, guvacine, and guvacoline are four major alkaloids in Areca nut.

13. b. Betel quid itself, with or without tobacco, has been identified as a group I carcinogen by the International Agency for Research on Cancer (IARC). Areca nut used in any form causes oral cancer in humans. Cancers of the esophagus, liver, pancreas, larynx, and lungs are also common among areca nut chewers. Chewing areca nut is considered the single most important etiological factor for developing OSF.
14. c. Pharmacological interventions are established for areca nut use disorders. Educational interventions focused on prevention and providing knowledge related to the harms and effects of betel nuts, aimed at enhancing awareness, and were found to have a positive impact. Psychological interventions included were mainly group-based, using techniques like cognitive behavior intervention and culturally tailored behavior change interventions (BCIs), adapted from smoking cessation programs. Only initial evidence of the efficacy of pharmacological treatment in areca nut use disorders was found in patients with depressive disorders.
15. c. Areca nut is helpful for patients with type 2 diabetes and prevents metabolic syndrome. It contains arecoline, an alkaloid that stimulates various brain receptors, promoting physical dependence and is associated with both stimulant and anxiolytic effects. It can cause or worsen conditions such as myocardial infarction, cardiac arrhythmias, hepatotoxicity, asthma, obesity, type 2 diabetes, metabolic syndrome, hypothyroidism, infertility, and adverse reproductive outcomes. Areca nut use (areca with or without tobacco) remains an orphan addiction with little research.

Caffeine

16. d. Smokers seem to metabolize caffeine slowly. Metabolism of caffeine essentially takes place in the liver through the cytochrome P450 pathway, especially CYP1A2. Certain medications, such as disulfiram or quinolones, have been shown to impair caffeine metabolism and prolong caffeine half-life through CYL1A2 inhibition. During pregnancy, the half-life of caffeine increases. Smokers metabolize caffeine more quickly through the acceleration of demethylation steps.
17. b. Thebaine; caffeine is metabolized in the liver into 10% theobromine, 4% theophylline, and 80% paraxanthine.
18. d. Caffeine use disorder is included in substance-related and addictive disorders. DSM-5 includes the following diagnoses related to caffeine: caffeine intoxication, caffeine withdrawal, other caffeine-induced disorders (e.g., anxiety and sleep disorders), and unspecified caffeine-related disorders. Caffeine use disorder is included in emerging measures and models.
19. d. Decreased appetite; diagnosis of caffeine withdrawal in ICD-10 includes lethargy and fatigue, psychomotor retardation or agitation, craving for stimulant drugs, increased appetite, insomnia or hypersomnia, bizarre or unpleasant dreams.
20. c. Both; other caffeine-induced disorders in DSM-5 include caffeine-induced anxiety disorders and caffeine-induced sleep disorders.
21. d. Caffeine is included under stimulants. Disorders due to the use of caffeine in ICD-11 include a single episode of harmful use of caffeine, harmful pattern of use of caffeine, caffeine intoxication, caffeine withdrawal, and caffeine-induced disorders, and it is not included under stimulants.

22. c. Caffeine is considered a doping substance controlled by the WADA. In humans, the regular consumption of coffee has been clearly linked to a decrease in the incidence of type 2 diabetes (Huxley et al. 2009). Caffeine influences the metabolism of uric acid and occurrence of gout (Choi et al.) Coffee (at a dosage of 300 mg caffeine per day) has been shown to protect against Parkinson's disease, with a risk reduction of 25% (Costa et al. 2010). Caffeine was considered a doping substance controlled by the WADA but was removed in 2004 from the list.
23. d. Gastric lavage should always be considered. Cardiovascular or neurologic toxicities occur frequently. Sinus tachycardia occurs but does not usually need any intervention unless there is an arrhythmia. Dialysis or hemofiltration may be necessary for extremely high caffeine levels. Gastric lavage is rarely done because of aspiration risk and should not be considered unless in <1 hour after intake.
24. c. Tolerance; a problematic pattern of caffeine use leading to clinically significant impairment or distress, as manifested by at least the first three of the following criteria occurring within a 12-month period: (1) A persistent desire or unsuccessful efforts to cut down or control caffeine use; (2) continued caffeine use despite knowledge of having a persistent or recurrent physical or psychological problem that is likely to have been caused or exacerbated by caffeine; (3) withdrawal, as manifested by either of the following: (i) the characteristic withdrawal syndrome for caffeine; (ii) caffeine (or a closely related) substance is taken to relieve or avoid withdrawal symptoms.
25. d. Analgesics are contraindicated. Caffeine withdrawal is self-limited, so a wait-and-see approach is privileged. Apart from general interventions such as rest, physical activity, and good fluid and electrolyte supply, in case of severe headaches, simple analgesia (e.g., paracetamol) can be used.

New Psychoactive Substances

26. d. These are safer for consumption than illicit drugs. The safety profile of NPS is still not completely understood and is a matter of debate.
27. c. These are not controlled by the United Nations drug conventions. These substances were developed in recent decades and do not fall under the schedules of the UN conventions of 1961, 1971, or 1988. Also (a) is incorrect because not all these substances are synthetic; let us recall plant-based NPSs such as ayahuasca and magic mushrooms.
28. b. Phenethylamines; these are a class of drugs with documented psychoactive and stimulant effects. Amphetamine, methamphetamine, and MDMA are phenethylamines controlled under the 1971 Convention of Psychotropic Substances.
29. c. NMDA agonists; psychedelics are agonists at 5HT2A receptors and antagonists at NMDARs
30. c. 1-benzylpiperazine (BZP); this was developed as an antiparasitic agent but is misused as a stimulant.
31. d. All of the above
32. a. Amphetamine-type stimulants; these were the only NPS included in the magnitude of substance use in India survey, 2019, with the explanation that data for other NPS is even more scarce. Another recent newspaper article-based study revealed similar findings.

33. b. Pharmacological effects and interactions are largely understood. Contrary to popular belief, the effects of plant-based substances are better understood as compared to synthetic NPS.
34. a. Anxiety and panic-like symptoms
35. c. MDMA was granted "Breakthrough Therapy" designation by the United States FDA) in 2017 for a development program for MDMA for the treatment of PTSD.
36. a. 0.4%
37. b. The intranasal form of esketamine, the S-enantiomer of racemic ketamine, was approved by the US FDA in 2019 for TRD in adults.

Drug Use in Special Populations

38. b. 1.3—the prevalence of current alcohol use in those between 10 and 17 years is 1.3%.
39. a. Obstetrics and gynecology—the T-ACE screening instrument is commonly used as a screening tool for high-risk drinking among pregnant women.
40. d. Macrocephaly—macrocephaly is not a feature of fetal alcohol syndrome.
41. b. 1.2%—the prevalence of inhalant use disorders in adolescents is 0.09%.
42. a. Nicotine replacement therapy—this is the pharmacological treatment of choice for childhood nicotine dependence.

United Nations Drug Conventions

43. d. Cambodia—Cambodia is not a part of the Golden Triangle.
44. a. Vienna—The secretariat of the INCB is located in Vienna.
45. d. It laid down an enforceable multilateral treaty—the First International Opium Convention did not lay down an enforceable multilateral treaty.
46. c. The Single Convention on Narcotic Drugs, 1961 contains 51 articles.
47. b. It was adopted in Geneva, Switzerland, in 1971—This statement regarding the Convention on Psychotropic Substances 1971 is false.
48. d. It is a quasi-judicial body—the statement regarding the INCB being a quasi-judicial body is false.
49. b. Schedule II—MDMA; MDMA is subsumed under Schedule I.
50. d. UNODC
51. b. Works with UNODC to eradicate hunger in vulnerable populations; the aim of the World Food Programme is to work with UNODC to eradicate hunger in vulnerable populations.
52. b. Etizolam—It was added to Schedule IV of the Convention on Psychotropic Substances of 1971 in 2020.

Historical Aspects of Substance Use

53. c. Turkey; it was first introduced to China by Turkish and Arab traders in the late sixth or early seventh century CE.
54. b. 1799.
55. c. North America.
56. b. *Cannabis brasiliensis*; all other species are cultivated for their yield of THC.

Miscellaneous

57. b. Maharashtra. Gujarat, Bihar, Nagaland, Mizoram, and Lakshadweep are dry states in India.
58. a. 30 mg/100 mL of blood.
59. b. Madagascar.
60. d. India; as of 2019, the Prohibition of Electronic Cigarettes (Production, Manufacture, Import, Export, Transport, Sale, Distribution, Storage and Advertisement) Act was passed in India.
61. c. Holi and Shiv Ratri are commonly associated with bhang intake in India.
62. b. Unexplained fever

Narcotic Drugs and Psychotropic Substances Act

63. c. Ministry of Finance; NDPS act is administered by the Ministry of Finance, Department of Revenue. Matters related to drug demand reduction are handled by the Ministry of Health and Family Welfare and the Ministry of Social Justice and Empowerment.
64. d. November 14, 1985
65. b. Article 47; if the Constitution of India directs the State to raise the level of nutrition and the standard of living and to improve public health as among its primary duties and in particular, the State shall endeavor to bring about the prohibition of intoxicating drinks and drugs which are injurious to health.
66. d. Poppy seeds; Seeds of *Papaver somniferum* are called the poppy seeds, while the latex that oozes out and dries is called the opium gum. Opium gum is the source of several alkaloids and drugs of abuse, while poppy seeds are not narcotic and are used as a condiment in Indian cooking.
67. d. Buprenorphine; ENDs include morphine, methadone, hydrocodone, oxycodone, codeine, fentanyl. Buprenorphine is a psychotropic.
68. d. Section 64a; immunity from prosecution to addicts volunteering for treatment states that any addict, who is charged with an offence punishable under Section 27 or with offences involving small quantity of narcotic drugs or psychotropic substances, who voluntarily seeks to undergo medical treatment for de-addiction from a hospital or an institution maintained or recognized by the government or a local authority and undergoes such treatment shall not be liable to prosecution under Section 27 or under any other section for offences involving small quantity of narcotic drugs or psychotropic substances: Provided that the said immunity from prosecution may be withdrawn if the addict does not undergo the complete treatment for de-addiction.
69. c. 2004; NDPS Act was amended in 1989, 2001, and 2014.
70. c. Methadone is classified as a narcotic.
71. a. Bhang; it is not included in the NDPS Act and is available legally in India.
72. d. All of the above; NDPS act applies to all citizens of India, including those outside India; and to all persons on ships and aircrafts registered in India, wherever they may be.
73. c. Can be both; penalty for possession of 1 kg of ganja, i.e., small quantity, includes rigorous imprisonment for up to 1 year or a fine up to ₹ 10,000 or both. First-time offenders also face a penalty.

74. d. All of the above; Section 39: Power of court to release certain offenders on probation
    a. When any addict is found guilty of an offence punishable under section 27 1(or for offences relating to small quantity of any narcotic drug or psychotropic substance) and if the court by which he is found guilty is of the opinion, regard being had to the age, character, antecedents or physical or mental condition of the offender, that it is expedient so to do, then, notwithstanding anything contained in this Act or any other law for the time being in force, the court may, instead of sentencing him at once to any imprisonment, with his consent, direct that he be released for undergoing medical treatment for detoxification or de-addiction from a hospital or an institution maintained or recognized by Government and on his entering into a bond in the form prescribed by the Central Government, with or without sureties, to appear and furnish before the court within a period not exceeding 1 year, a report regarding the result of his medical treatment and in the meantime, to abstain from the commission of any offence under Chapter IV.
    b. If it appears to the court, having regard to the report regarding the result of the medical treatment furnished under subsection (1), that it is expedient to do so, the court may direct the release of the offender after due admonition on his entering into a bond in the form prescribed by the Central Government, with or without sureties, for abstaining from the commission of any offence under Chapter IV during such period not exceeding 3 years as the court may deem fit to specify or on his failure so to abstain, to appear before the court and receive sentence when called upon during such period.
75. The responsibilities of the OIC of an RMI in relation to ENDs is to ensure:
    a. ENDs shall be dispensed to selected patients registered with RMI
    b. RMI uses ENDs in a licit manner
    c. The stock of ENDs in RMI is uninterrupted and adequately available (3 months stock)
    d. ENDs kept under safe custody
    e. Record of Form 3 E for each patient to be kept for 2 years from the date of last entry
76. d. Haryana; the Central Bureau of Narcotics licenses farmers to cultivate opium poppy in the notified tracts of Uttar Pradesh, Madhya Pradesh, and Rajasthan. Such cultivation is only on the Central Government account.
77. a. All IDUs must be compulsorily de-addicted. IDUs among the inmates of prisons shall be compulsorily de-addicted, and they shall not be given supplied clean needles and syringes and allowed to inject drugs. They shall also not be supplied oral buprenorphine or methadone for abuse as substitutes.

Drug De-Addiction Programme of India

78. a. 1988
79. b. Ministry of Social Justice and Empowerment
80. a. NDDTC, AIIMS New Delhi—The National Nodal Centre for DDAP is the National Drug Dependence Treatment Centre, All India Institute of Medical Sciences, New Delhi.

81. b. Ministry of Social Justice and Empowerment—Nasha Mukt Bharat Abhiyan under DDAP is implemented by the Ministry of Social Justice and Empowerment.
82. d. Providing evidence-based treatment is not an objective of the DDAP.

National Aids Control Programme

83. c. 20 times; PWID are estimated to be 22 times more likely than the general population to be living with HIV.
84. b. Uttar Pradesh
85. b. 10%; HIV prevalence rates among PWID were 9.9%, as per the survey.
86. d. Children of people living with HIV
87. a. >1 per 100,000 exposures
88. d. Rehabilitation and community reintegration
89. c. Less than 100% exchange
90. b. Buprenorphine
91. c. 95–95–95: 95% of the population tested for HIV, 95% of those found positive on ART, and 95% of those showing viral load suppression
92. d. Family members of PWID

Drug-Related Laws and Policies—International Scenario

93. b. Nixon
94. c. MORE Act of 2022 stands for Marijuana Opportunity Reinvestment and Expungement Act.
95. a. The iron law of prohibition is a term coined by Richard Cowan in 1986, which posits that as law enforcement becomes more intense, the potency of prohibited substances increases.
96. d. Harm reduction practices normalize drug use in the society.
97. c. Safe injection sites

Case-Based Scenarios

98. b. 3 hours
    It is known that 30 mL of whiskey contains approximately 10 g of pure ethanol. In ideal conditions, the liver metabolizes 10 g of ethanol in 1 hour. Thus, 30 g of ethanol will be metabolized in 3 hours.
99. c. Juvenile Justice Act; the person will be convicted under IPC Section 506 (1) for criminal intimidation and Section 77 of the Juvenile Justice Act (giving intoxicating liquor, narcotic drugs, or psychotropic substances to a child).
100. a. Stabilize vitals, reassure, send urine for toxicology screening, and maintain a calm environment. The patient's symptoms appear consistent with ingestion of a hallucinogen such as LSD or psilocybin, the effects of which wear off with time. Thus, symptomatic management along with prevention of harm to self and others are the mainstay of immediate management.

FURTHER READING

1. Ambedkar A, Agarwal A, Rao R, Mishra AK, Khandelwal SK, Chadha RK on behalf of the group of investigators for the National Survey on Extent and Pattern of Substance Use in India. Magnitude of Substance Use in India. New Delhi: Ministry of Social Justice and Empowerment, Government of India; 2019.
2. Athukorala IA, Tilakaratne WM, Jayasinghe RD. Areca Nut Chewing: Initiation, Addiction, and Harmful Effects Emphasizing the Barriers and Importance of Cessation. J Addict. 2021;2021:9967097.
3. Chakma JK, Kumar H, Bhargava S, Khanna T. The e-cigarettes ban in India: an important public health decision. Lancet. 2020;5(8):E426.
4. Choi HK, Willett W, Curhan G. Coffee consumption and risk of incident gout in men: a prospective study. Arthritis Rheum. 2007;56:2049-55.
5. Chopra R N, Chopra I C. (1955). Quasi-medical Use of Opium in India and Its Effects. [online] Available from https://www.unodc.org/unodc/en/data-and-analysis/bulletin/bulletin_1955-01-01_3_page002.html#s0007 [Last accessed December, 2023].
6. Commissionerate Transport, Government of Assam. Rules against Drunk Driving Cases. [online] Available from https://comtransport.assam.gov.in/frontimpotentdata/rules-against-drunk-driving-cases [Last accessed December, 2023].
7. Dhingra K, Jhanjee S. A Review of Intervention Strategies for Areca Nut Use Cessation. Indian J Psychol Med. 2023;45(2):117-23. https://doi.org/10.1177/02537176221144711
8. El-Guebaly N, Carrà G, Galanter M, Baldacchino AM, editors. Textbook of Addiction Treatment: International Perspectives. Switzerland: Springer International Publishing; 2021.
9. Ganesan K, Rahman S, Zito PM. Anabolic Steroids.In: StatPearls [Internet]. Treasure Island (FL): StatPearls Publishing; 2023.
10. Gupta PC, Warnakulasuriya S. Global epidemiology of areca nut usage. Addict Biol. 2002;7(1):77-83.
11. Hansen C, Alas H, Davis E Jr. (2023). Where Is Marijuana Legal? A Guide to Marijuana Legalization. [online] Available from https://www.usnews.com/news/best-states/articles/where-is-marijuana-legal-a-guide-to-marijuana-legalization [Last accessed December, 2023].
12. Harm reduction: An approach to reducing risky health behaviours in adolescents. Paediatr Child Health. 2008 Jan;13(1):53-60.
13. Hayes JP. The Opium Wars in China. [online] Available from https://asiapacificcurriculum.ca/learning-module/opium-wars-china#:~:text=The%20Chinese%20government%20recognized%20that,of%20beating%20offenders%20100%20times [Last accessed December, 2023].
14. History of Tobacco. [online] Available from https://www.afro.who.int/sites/default/files/2017-09/Chapter%2032.%20The%20history%20of%20tobacco.pdf [Last accessed December, 2023].
15. Hwang KAJ, Saadabadi A. Lysergic Acid Diethylamide (LSD). In: StatPearls [Internet]. Treasure Island (FL): StatPearls Publishing; 2023.
16. Karpinski JP, Timpe EM, Lubsch L. Smoking cessation treatment for adolescents. J Pediatr Pharmacol Ther. 2010;15(4):249-63.

17. Kathiresan P, Sarkar S. Club Drugs in India: An Analysis of Newspaper Reports. Indian J Psychol Med. 2022;44(3):311-3.
18. Marijuana Policy Project. The MORE Act. [online] Available from https://www.mpp.org/policy/federal/the-more-act/ [Last accessed December, 2023].
19. Ministry of Social Justice and Empowerment, Government of India. (2019). Magnitude of Substance Use in India. Executive Summary. [online] Available from https://static.pib.gov.in/WriteReadData/userfiles/Exec-Sum_For%20Media.pdf [Last accessed December, 2023].
20. Mosher CJ, and Akins S. Drugs and drug policy: The control of consciousness alteration. SAGE Publications, 2007. Inc., https://doi.org/10.4135/9781452224763.
21. Murphy M, Eske J. (2023). What are the odds of getting HIV? [online] Available from https://www.medicalnewstoday.com/articles/chances-of-getting-hiv#summary-table [Last accessed December, 2023].
22. Nadkarni A, Tu A, Garg A, Gupta D, Gupta S, Bhatia U, et al. Alcohol use among adolescents in India: a systematic review. Global Mental Health. Cambridge: Cambridge University Press; 2022. pp. 1-25.
23. National AIDS Control Organisation, Ministry of Health and Family Welfare. (2017). National Strategic Plan for HIV/AIDS and STI 2017 2024. Paving the Way for an AIDS Free India. [online] Available from https://naco.gov.in/sites/default/files/Paving%20the%20Way%20for%20an%20AIDS%2015122017.pdf [Last accessed December, 2023].
24. National AIDS Control Organization. National Integrated Biological and Behavioral Surveillance (IBBS), India 2014-15. New Delhi: NACO, Ministry of Health and Family Welfare, Government of India; 2015.
25. Patanè FG, Liberto A, Maria Maglitto AN, Malandrino P, Esposito M, Amico F, et al. Nandrolone Decanoate: Use, Abuse and Side Effects. Medicina (Kaunas). 2020;56(11):606.
26. Patel V. The politics of alcoholism in India. BMJ. 1998;316(7141):1394A.
27. Piacentino D, Kotzalidis GD, Del Casale A, Aromatario MR, Pomara C, Girardi P, Sani G. Anabolic-androgenic steroid use and psychopathology in athletes. A systematic review. Curr Neuropharmacol. 2015;13(1):101-21.
28. Sapkota A, Khurshid H, Qureshi IA, Jahan N, Went TR, Sultan W, Alfonso M. Efficacy and Safety of Intranasal Esketamine in Treatment-Resistant Depression in Adults: A Systematic Review. Cureus. 2021;13(8):e17352.
29. Sarkar S, Bhatia G, Dhawan A. Clinical Practice Guidelines for Assessment and Management of Patients with Substance Intoxication Presenting to the Emergency Department. Indian J Psychiatry. 2023;65(2):196-211.
30. Scott-Ham M, Stark MM. (2016). Substance Misuse: Legal Highs. [online] Available from https://doi.org/10.1016/B978-0-12-800034-2.00354-2 [Last accessed December, 2023].
31. Smith KW, Sicignano DJ, Hernandez AV, White CM. MDMA-Assisted Psychotherapy for Treatment of Posttraumatic Stress Disorder: A Systematic Review with Meta-Analysis. J Clin Pharmacol. 2022;62(4):463-71.
32. The Editors of Encyclopaedia Britannica. (2023). Cannabis. [online] Available from https://www.britannica.com/plant/cannabis-plant [Last accessed December, 2023].

33. The Editors of Encyclopaedia Britannica. (2023). Opium Trade. British and Chinese History. [online] Available from https://www.britannica.com/money/topic/opium-trade [Last accessed December, 2023].
34. The Editors of Encyclopaedia Britannica. War on Drugs. [online] Available from https://www.britannica.com/topic/war-on-drugs [Last accessed December, 2023].
35. Tilakaratne WM, Klinikowski MF, Saku T, Peters TJ, Warnakulasuriya S. Oral submucous fibrosis: review on aetiology and pathogenesis. Oral Oncol. 2006;42(6):561-8.
36. United Nations Office on Drugs and Crime. (2020). Drug Use and Health Consequences. World Drug Report, 2020. [online] Available from https://wdr.unodc.org/wdr2020/field/WDR20_Booklet_2.pdf [Last accessed December, 2023].
37. United Nations Office on Drugs and Crime. (2023). The Synthetic Drug Phenomenon. Contemporary Issues on Drugs. World Drug Report. [online] Available from https://www.unodc.org/res/WDR-2023/WDR23_B3_CH1_Synthetic_drugs.pdf [Last accessed December, 2023].
38. United Nations Office on Drugs and Crime. Phenethylamines. [online] Available from https://www.unodc.org/LSS/SubstanceGroup/Details/275dd468-75a3-4609-9e96-cc5a2f0da467 [Last accessed December, 2023].
39. United States Office Drugs and Crime. (2023). Recent Developments Involving Psychedelics. Contemporary Issues on Drugs. World Drug Report. [online] Available from https://www.unodc.org/res/WDR-2023/WDR23_B3_CH2_psychedelics.pdf [Last accessed December, 2023].
40. van Elk M, Yaden DB. Pharmacological, neural, and psychological mechanisms underlying psychedelics: A critical review. Neurosci Biobehav Rev. 2022;140:104793.
41. World Health Organization, Regional Office for South-East Asia. (2010). Report on people who inject drugs in the South-East Asia Region. WHO Regional Office for South-East Asia. [online] Available from https://apps.who.int/iris/handle/10665/206320 [Last accessed December, 2023].
42. Zanos P, Gould TD. Mechanisms of ketamine action as an antidepressant. Mol Psychiatry. 2018;23(4):801-11.